Eat No Evil
Cookbook

Colleen A. Sundermeyer, Ph.D.
Velma L. Sundermeyer, R.N.

Eat No Evil Cookbook

New Outlook Publishing
6373 Riverside Boulevard
Box 114
Sacramento, CA 95831

Printed in the United States of America

ISBN 0-9621928-1-3

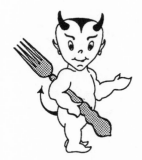

About the Authors

Dr. Colleen A. Sundermeyer, author of two books, *Emotional Weight* and *Eat No Evil Cookbook*, holds a master's degree in psychology and a doctorate in nutrition. She has been published in numerous newspapers, and has been a guest on radio and television programs across the country.

In addition to writing, Colleen also provides lectures to corporations nationwide. In her book *Emotional Weight*, Colleen's expertise and sincere interest in understanding eating problems has helped countless people. Now, people can also enjoy her unique cookbook, which has an educational focus, along with terrific tasting recipes for people on the go.

Velma L. Sundermeyer, author of *Eat No Evil Cookbook*, is a registered nurse and a mother of three, and lives in Ohio. Her collection of delicious recipes started in 1955 when her husband John joined the Air Force. While living in rural England, Velma started her cooking adventure on a small one burner stove.

Having always enjoyed a challenge, she focused on preparing well balanced meals for her family, and always had enough for unexpected visitors eager for a good meal. Velma's experiences are reflected in her recipes. They are all easy-to-follow practical recipes for lifetime health and vitality.

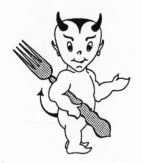

Acknowledgements

Many thanks go to Sharon Ray for her expert editing, typesetting and page layout, and to Jon Lewis for his proofreading and overall production guidance. Without their special care, hard work and insight, this book could not have become a reality. Also, this book wouldn't be what it is without our cute little devil and the creative artistry and cover design of Mark Sandell. A special word of thanks to Mark Sundermeyer for inspiring the name *Eat No Evil*. Last, but never least, we would like to thank those courageous people who have volunteered their taste buds for our cooking experiments. Bon Appetit!

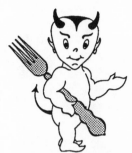

Contents

Eat No Evil
Cookbook

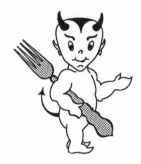

1. Introduction

"Yes indeed...Home Sweet Home! Gosh, I'm hungry. Hmmm...what's to eat? Now, what in the world is that? Ugh! Could it be one of the kids' science projects?" Most everyone at some time has had an unidentified object in their refrigerator. We wrote this cookbook hoping to make life a little easier -- and to fill your kitchen with more pleasant encounters.

We want you to kick off your shoes -- of course, not in the kitchen -- and prepare to have a good time! You can put your mind to rest and enjoy how easy we've made cooking these delicious meals.

Home shouldn't be just a pit stop and a convenient place to sleep and wash clothes. Fill your home with wonderful aromatic smells that could arouse distant neighbors and pets! Believe it or not, cooking can be enjoyable. We want to introduce you to your stove and refrigerator, pots and pans -- and hundreds of great tasting recipes. We want you to have a devil of a good time!

In writing this book we felt strongly about the idea that there is no such thing as a bad, evil or forbidden food. THAT'S RIGHT! And springing up quite unexpectedly is our fun-loving little devil, who serves as a reminder to relax and enjoy cooking! Nowhere in this book do we discuss diets or calorie counting. Simply relax.

We would like young people just beginning to cook for a family to become food wise and learn moderation. How much better off their children will be.

We have taken the guesswork out of cooking with our upbeat collection of over 200 healthful recipes used time after time, and ideas designed to make cooking fun, nutritious and kitchen-efficient in an easy-to-read format.

There is no need to panic in the kitchen. *Eat No Evil* will tell you everything you want to know -- from fascinating bits of trivia, to creative snacks, to which herbs and spices and side dishes fit best for great taste. You can whip up delicious meals quickly and inexpensively with our money saving tip section. We even have a recipe section for kids.

And recognizing that even the most skilled cooks make mistakes, we've also included a devilishly funny section on how to creatively use mistakes when all seems lost.

Stop worrying. Stop counting calories. Stop depriving yourself and start enjoying great food. You'll have a devil of a good time.

Bon appetit!

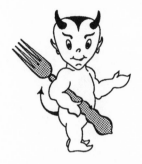

2. There is No Such Thing as a Bad, Evil, or Forbidden Food

The philosophy of the *Eat No Evil Cookbook* is that there are no bad, evil or forbidden foods. All food should be eaten to moderation. Therefore, we decided not to eliminate fats, sugars, eggs, salt, and countless other foods people have labelled bad or forbidden. Instead, we have chosen to reduce rather than eliminate these foods. By reducing, we are achieving moderation. All foods, when eaten in moderation, supply our bodies with vital life-sustaining nutrients. For people on sodium- and/or cholesterol-restricted programs we have included a Food Substitute Chart. Keep in mind however, that moderation has been used in all our recipes already.

The next time you are eating, take the time to notice how you have labeled that food. Have you called it a bad or forbidden food? Did you then eat more out of guilt? Instead of eliminating the food -- eliminate your attitude toward that food. All food can be eaten, if eaten in moderation. Once you become skilled in the kitchen, preparing food will be a cinch! There is no need to devour an entire cheesecake.

There will always be another cheesecake. *Eat No Evil* is an educational book, filled with interesting cooking trivia, as well as reference charts on Herbs, Food Substitution, Complementary Side Dishes, a Table of Equivalents, Money Saving Ideas, and a chart on Keeping Food Safe and Fresh. We want you to become food wise and forget the calorie counting. Each chapter has a brief introduction that will help you learn new skills and gain confidence in trying new recipes. We even have a Kids' Recipe section and a Vegetarian section.

Because even the most skilled cooks make mistakes, we included a devilishly funny section on how to creatively use mistakes -- not throw them out! Mistakes sometimes end up producing some of our best meals. The secret is not to panic -- you can always order a pizza! With every recipe we will give you some complementary side dishes. We also included a chart you can use in conjunction with other cookbooks. We hope our recipes and suggestions will be useful tools in your kitchen.

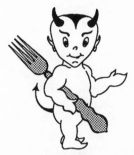

3. Read the Label

We want you to become food wise, not food restrictive. Have you ever read a label and said "What is that stuff?" Start asking yourself, "How can that food sit on the shelf for three years and not spoil?" What is artificial chocolate flavoring? -- yuk! Most of the popular soft drinks are high in sugar, sodium, and phosphorus, and have a long shelf life. It is the phosphoric acid that is added to hold the sugar in suspension so it will not crystallize that gives it a long shelf life. There is nothing wrong with phosphoric acid, sodium, or sugar in soft drinks consumed in moderation. Pop is something most people overuse, especially if it says, "only one calorie." Too much pop can cause loss of calcium from the body. Even meats, chocolate, and caffeine contain phosphoric acid and cause depletion of calcium stores. Too much sugar also causes calcium losses.

Becoming a label reader is another way to take care of your body.

As you begin to introduce new foods into your eating plan, read labels on the foods you purchase, or you're getting ripped off! When you're not food wise, you're being robbed of nutrients, your health, and your money! Buy foods that don't have a long list of ingredients, such as fresh fruits and vegetables. There is no list of ingredients that comes on an apple or a carrot stick!

Bread, for example, starts out as a highly nutritious food until it is refined and the bran and wheat germ are taken out. All that is left is the endosperm (starch) and a more expensive bread because of the process. It is also bleached to look a pretty white color. When bread is refined, it loses 22 nutrients; through an enrichment process, only three B vitamins, vitamin D, calcium, and iron are replaced. I hardly call this a fair exchange of nutrients!

Items are not always what they appear on the label, and all substances in a food product don't have to be listed on the label, which can be misleading. A food that states "no salt" could still have sodium. The word "light" could be referring to the color and not its caloric content, and if you don't read the label you'll fall hook, line, and sinker! The words "sugar free" don't mean it is lower in calories; it may still have artificial or non-nutritive sweetener added.

Another example of how misleading advertising can be is the labeling of fat content. It may sound good to you if you see hot dogs labeled as "95% fat free" (by weight). But you are not interested in how much the fat weighs. You want to know how many of the hot dogs' calories come from that fat. That would be about 50-80%, since fat has a lot more calories than do carbohydrates or protein. For food to be truly "low fat," fat should not comprise more than 25% of the food's total *calories*, not its weight.

Let's say a label states that a food contains 550 calories per serving and 35 grams of fat per serving. What does that tell you? Nothing -- until you do a simple calculation to see if the food is more than 25% fat. Since fat has 9 calories per gram, multiply the number of grams of fat (also listed on the label) by 9. For example, if the product has 35 grams of fat, 9 x 35 = 315 calories of fat. Then divide the calories of fat (315) by the calories per serving (550). This gives you 0.57, which when multiplied by 100 to get a percentage equals 57%. Therefore 57% of that food's total calories come from fat, and it could not be classified, and should not be thought of, as a low fat food.

All products labeled "low calorie," "reduced calorie," "diet" or "dietetic" fall under the FDA (Food and Drug Administration) and must contain no more than 40 calories or have at least one-third fewer calories than the regular product of that type. If a product is labeled "enriched" or "fortified" it means vitamins and minerals and/or protein have been added, and the product must have nutrients labeled. If the word "imitation" appears on the label, it means the product is nutritionally inferior to the real thing. The word "natural" doesn't mean anything, unless used on meats and poultry labeling, because the FDA has no regulations on the word "natural." We're sure you are realizing why it is important to become food wise. Even the word "naturally flavored" holds no guarantee that artificial colors, additives, or preservatives have not been added. Just because it says "one calorie" doesn't make it a perfect food!

The USDA (United States Department of Agriculture) has no regulations on the word "organic." Labels indicating that the product is sugarless or sugar-free mean that it can't contain sucrose (table sugar), but it can contain other sweeteners, like fructose, honey, syrup, sorbitol, and mannitol.

Even mineral water has no regulation on it, and could be regular tap water with minerals added. Lastly, when buying bread, wheat bread is really the same as white bread. You want to buy *whole wheat* bread, and "whole wheat" should be the first ingredient listed. Take your time and make good choices for yourself. It's *your* body. Take a shopping list with you, so you don't get frustrated trying to remember every-thing and then just grab anything off the shelf! If you like to eat frozen dinners, which are usually nutritionally incomplete in calcium and B vitamins as well as fiber, add to the dinner a salad or some brown rice or whole wheat bread to increase the nutrient value. Once you start taking your time, you'll realize that the chunk tuna you've been buying is more expensive than the flaked tuna, and mackerel is less expensive than salmon or tuna.

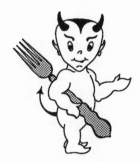

4. Spice It Up

Cooking Trivia: Herbs

You can keep your herbs and spices 6-9 months if you keep them dry.

The flavor of herbs and spices is enhanced when they are cooked or soaked in stock, oil, lemon juice, vinegar, or butter.

You can add herbs or spices to soups 30 minutes before serving or right away if you like a lot of flavor.

When using herbs, 1/3 teaspoon of ground herbs or 1 teaspoon of dried herbs is equal in strength to 1 tablespoon of fresh herbs.

Saffron is so expensive because it takes 75,000 crocus flowers to produce 1 pound of saffron.

It is important to keep herbs dry. Basil will turn black and most herbs get musty and lose their flavor.

Fresh herbs can be kept in a jar of water for about 4-5 days, whereas drying herbs allows you to keep them for 6-9 months.

Most herbs can be frozen and then used right from the freezer in soups, sauces, and vegetable dishes.

Cayenne is high in vitamin C and is rumored to contain several medicinal properties.

Parsley is useful in eliminating garlic and onion breath.

Tarragon can never be grown from seeds, but must be started from cuttings or bought as a small plant.

Seasoning with Herbs and Spices

Let's give your salt and pepper shaker a rest and venture into some terrific new flavors. Herbs and spices should be no mystery. You'll be amazed at how herbs and spices enhance the natural flavor of food rather than masking its flavor. We want you to use herbs and spices for everyday cooking.

In no time at all you'll become familiar with the different tastes and textures and confidently add...a touch of oregano, a dash of rosemary, a pinch of basil and -- presto! You can make foods exciting again! Now the only problem is to remember the next time what herbs and spices you used. Don't worry, that's why we wrote this book.

Let us first explain the difference between herbs and spices. Herbs are from the leaves of low growing annual or perennial plants that grow in temperate climates. Some of the most popular herbs are basil, oregano, thyme, sage, parsley, savory, bay leaf, marjoram, rosemary, mint, and chervil. Spices include cinnamon, ginger, and nutmeg. They come from tropical barks, roots, or fruits, or berries of perennial shrubs. Seeds such as dill, caraway, and fennel are from annual plants. Garlic powder, onion powder, cayenne, chili powder, and paprika are examples of dehydrated vegetables.

The flavor of herbs and spices is enhanced when they are cooked or soaked in or with lemon juice, vinegar, or butter. Keep in mind that you can add your herbs to soups 30 minutes before the dish is finished or right at the start if you like a lot of flavor. You can keep herbs and spices for 6-9 months, if you keep them dry.

Stronger flavored herbs and seeds should be used sparingly. Examples are oregano, rosemary, thyme, sage, fennel seed, tarragon, and savory. Some of our favorite herbs are thyme (which all of us could use more of), basil, and savory, which are all members of the mint family.

Any combination of herbs, spices, seeds, and dehydrated vegetables can be considered a seasoning blend. You can use single herbs and spices or choose a seasoning combination, like poultry seasoning, curry powder, chili powder, or allspice -- or even make your own seasoning creation.

Try a little basil on your carrots, or try sprinkling a touch of ginger or curry on your chicken. Zucchini tastes wonderful sprinkled with basil, tarragon, and thyme. Dill and caraway have a similar taste and are delicious in breads. We often garnish fresh fruit with mint.

Herbs Are Easy to Grow

Herbs can be mixed easily right along with a flower garden. It's simple: as you cook you can pop outdoors, pinch or cut a few herbs, and then pop back into the kitchen and wash, dry, chop, and use.

The most important thing to remember when growing herbs is to keep the soil well-drained and, with the exception of mints, keep them in full sunlight. Most herbs can be started from seeds, or you can buy small plants at the nursery. You may not want a garden and may find small pots of herbs just right. A garden, however, may consist of one- to two-foot plots for each herb, which will keep you with a good supply of herbs for spring, summer, and autumn.

To harvest large amounts of herbs, try to choose them at their peak flavor, which is usually just before the flower. Don't worry after cutting. Mother nature will help them renew themselves.

Drying and Storing Herbs

There are many different ways to preserve herbs. We will tell you the easiest no-fuss way. First, you should cut long stems so you can tie them in bundles using fairly heavy string. Then hang them from nails in the garage or kitchen. Because thyme is a short plant you will need to cut it and place it in a mesh bag, and also hang it up. Are you thinking "Where do I get a mesh bag?" You can dry your herbs in the mesh bags that oranges and grapefruits come packaged in.

Direct heat drying is another idea that could be used with chives and parsley, which are more succulent. They can be washed and then dried in the microwave oven between layers of paper towels. The time depends on the oven power, so test every few minutes. You'll be able to tell when they are dry. Let the chives and parsley cool. Then place in a jar and cover. It's just that simple.

Herbs can also be dried by placing in a colander and then forcing them through the colander with a drinking glass or spoon. Once herbs are dried they should be kept in jars or bottles with tight-fitting caps, away from sunlight and in a dry, cool place. Don't forget to label them and keep them in your kitchen cabinet as they await their destiny.

Freezing Herbs

Yes, most herbs can be frozen. They first must be boiled for about 15 seconds, and then immersed in cold water for a minute. Dry between paper towels. Next, place several tablespoons of each herb in a plastic bag, and freeze. To use, simply add the frozen herbs to soups, vegetable dishes, or sauces.

Hot Stuff

There are certain kinds of seasonings that you shouldn't be too generous with, unless you have dinner guests you don't care much for. Your guests could leave your home feeling quite hot and bothered if you splash on too much cayenne and chili powder. These dehydrated vegetables are a blend of the hottest chili peppers around. Mustard seed is also sharp, hot, and very pungent. Paprika, another dehydrated vegetable, is the ground part of the sweet chili pepper.

Everyday Herb Chart

Included in all our recipes we have already selected the herbs we feel would work best. However, our Everyday Herb Chart is available for an easy reference when cooking with different recipes. Remember, we want to make your life in the kitchen a simple one.

Herbs, Spices, Seeds	How It Tastes	How It Is Used
Allspice	A blend of cinnamon, nutmeg, and cloves.	Fish, soups, fruitcakes, cookies, red and yellow vegetables.
Basil	Sweet and pungent flavor and is sometimes peppery.	Pesto, fish, eggs, tomatoes, pasta, stews, meats, salads, sauces.
Bay Leaf	Distinct aromatic, woody kind of flavor.	Lentils, poultry, eggs, soups, salads, chowders, marinades, artichokes, eggplant.
Chervil	Tasty parsley flavor.	Vegetables, cottage cheese, meats, figs, stews, salads, sauces, eggs.
Cinnamon	Spicy flavor, pleasant aroma.	Pastries, desserts, fruits, puddings, sweet potatoes, carrots, squash, beans.
Cloves	Spicy, hot.	Sweet pork, soups, desserts, potatoes, sauces, fruit, beans, carrots, squash.
Cumin	Sweet and salty taste.	Chili, fish, meatloaf, eggs, beans, cabbage, pies, cheeses.
Coriander	Slight lemon-orange flavor.	Cookies, pea soup, pastries, casseroles, cheeses, meats, Mexican dishes.
Curry	A combination of many spices; pleasant fragrant taste.	Soups, shellfish, poultry, creamed and scalloped potatoes, vegetables, meats, fruits.

Ginger	Sweet, spicy, and aromatic.	Cakes, pies, carrots, fruits, meats, yellow vegetables, beets, dressings.
Marjoram	Slight mint flavor; delicate.	Omelets, pork, lamb, beef, fish, vegetables, soups, chowders, stews.
Mint	Fruity, aromatic.	Lamb, veal, fish, fruit, sauces, carrots, cabbage, beans, potatoes.
Nutmeg	Spicy, sweet.	All kinds of desserts, vegetables, sauces, fruits, meats.
Oregano	Similar to thyme; stronger than marjoram.	Pizza, Italian, Mexican, meats, fish, vegetables, mushrooms, dips.
Rosemary	Refreshing, pungent, savory flavor.	Poultry, omelets, breads, sauces, marinades, vegetables, soups, fruits, stuffings, eggs.
Saffron	Pleasantly bittersweet.	Rice dishes, potatoes, fish, stews, sauces, soups, veal, chicken.
Sage	Pungent, long-lasting flavor.	Pork, lamb, veal, poultry, squash, stuffings, fish, salads, pumpkin, fish, dips, cream soups.
Savory	Aromatic, sage flavor.	Lentils, soups, salads, tomatoes, beets, peas.
Tarragon	Pleasant, licorice-anise flavor.	Eggs, fish, shellfish, poultry, vinegar, broccoli, cauliflower, soups, sauces.
Thyme	Pleasant clove flavor.	Fish, gumbo, tomatoes, soups, poultry, cheese sauces, onions, carrots, potatoes.

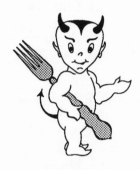

5. Meal Planning Ideas

Cooking Trivia: Everyday Fare

Keep cover off when cooking cabbage, brussels sprouts, or broccoli for a less sulfur-tasting vegetable.

If honey solidifies, place the whole jar in a saucepan of water and heat gently until it liquifies or cook in the microwave on low heat 1/2 to 1 minute.

Extra virgin olive oil is the best; it comes from the first pressing, whereas pure olive oil comes from the second pressing and has a more bitter flavor.

When bread is toasted, the starch converts to a sugar called dextrose -- and makes the bread taste sweeter.

Tamari sauce is a Japanese soy sauce; it has a better, richer flavor than the common Chinese soy sauce.

Bananas, avocado, pineapple, and melon do not store well in the refrigerator.

Olive oil is the best oil for salads, and peanut oil works great for wok cooking.

Adding an acid, like lemon, to wilted vegetables freshens them.

Some foods pop due to the skin or shell, such as sausages, hot dogs, white potatoes, and squash, so pierce the skin before cooking.

Clarified butter is pure butterfat with all the water and milk solids removed.

Wild rice is not a rice -- but the seed of a grass that grows in marshy areas.

Sugar and fat molecules attract microwaves and will cook faster.

Long grain rice cooks up fluffy, and short grain rice is soft and sticky.

By adding lemon juice to your fruit or salad, you can prevent browning or enzymatic decay.

Oil is used in low-cholesterol cheeses instead of milk fat.

White rice is polished with glucose to make it look whiter; it doesn't have the bran and germ or outer husk like brown rice.

Adding a dash of baking powder to your vegetables will make them bright and colorful.

When making a cream sauce, it is the heat that breaks down the starch molecules and causes thickening.

Add a little oil to rice to prevent foaming.

Minute rice and instant oatmeal need no cooking -- just warming up -- because they are pre-gelatinized starches.

Animal shortening is made from lard (fat from hogs) that is refined.

Diet margarine is 50% water, in comparison to spreads, which are 35% water and 60% fat. All margarines are fortified with vitamin A and have the same amount of nutrition as butter.

Salads made with fresh vegetables and vinegar and oil dressings keep well for several days in a covered container in the refrigerator.

Marinade type salads are great for serving large groups of people. They make large amounts and can be prepared ahead of time.

Don't use fresh pineapple, papaya or figs in gelatin salads. The enzyme bromelin breaks down the protein bonds and prevents the gelatin from jelling.

Pineapple is useful when baking ham. It acts as a tenderizer.

Try adding powdered or cubed chicken or beef bouillon to vegetables while they are cooking. Also add a pinch of your favorite herb or herbs.

The hardest part of cooking is deciding what to cook!

Useful Food Substitutes

Being creative and flexible with your cooking is part of having fun in the kitchen. This section will give you some useful substitutes for sugar, fat, eggs, and many other foods. We included this section not because any of these foods are bad, but as a way to give foods a slightly different flavor and texture.

If these substitutes are used for health reasons, that's fine -- or if you just want to try something different, that's fine too. Remember, moderation with all foods is our philosophy.

Included in all our recipes are useful food substitutes and just how much to use. We designed the chart to be used as a handy reference when making other recipes or creating your own. We want you to have fun and remain flexible. If this section makes you nervous, try reading our devilishly funny mistake section and realize that even the most skilled cooks make mistakes.

The average yield of our recipes is about 4 servings. It is easier to multiply recipes than to divide them. All the recipes in this book use Grade A "medium" eggs. Yogurt or sour half and half can be used in place of sour cream.

Honey is heavier than table sugar and has a higher liquid content. Therefore, to substitute honey for sugar, reduce the sweetener in the recipe by one-fourth and reduce the liquid in the recipe by one-eighth. Barley malt and rice syrup are also used as substitutes for table sugar. They are even heavier than honey, so when substituting these two grain syrups for table sugar you should reduce the sweetener in your recipe by one-half and reduce the liquid in the recipe by one-eighth.

Food Substitute Chart

Main Ingredient	*Substitute*
Whole milk	Evaporated milk, non-fat skim milk, buttermilk, soy milk, acidophilus milk.
One egg	1/4 cup egg substitute, 1 egg white, 2 Tablespoons baking powder and 1 teaspoon vegetable oil.
Two eggs	One egg and one egg white, 2 egg whites and 1 Tablespoon vegetable oil, 1/4 cup mashed tofu.
Butter	Mazola Extra Light Corn Oil Spread or Kraft Touch of Butter Spread, Canola oil, olive oil, safflower oil, peanut oil, corn oil, vegetable oil, sesame oil, or broth for sautéing or frying.
Sour cream	Plain yogurt, sour half and half, sour milk, plain Kefir (cultured milk).
Cream sauce	Use cornstarch, white flour, arrowroot flour, or Kuzu and mix with low fat milk. Use 2 teaspoons arrowroot in place of 1 Tablespoon cornstarch. Use 1-1/2 teaspoons arrowroot in place of 1 Tablespoon flour.

Chocolate	Carob (Use same amount as chocolate and 1 Tablespoon vegetable oil).
Unbleached white flour	Whole wheat, cake flour, pastry flour, whole wheat pastry flour (rye flour, rice flour, soy flour all need an addition of gluten flour to rise; approximately 1/4 cup).
Regular cheese	Low cholesterol cheese, low fat cheese, soy cheese.
Cream Cheese	Tofu.
Table sugar	Honey, barley malt, rice syrup, fruit juices. Reduce liquid by 1/4 cup in recipe.
Peanut butter	Almond butter, sesame tahini. Use same amount as peanut butter.
Jelly or jam	Apple or pear butter.
Whipped cream	Low fat milk (8 ounces mixed with 1/2 teaspoon cream of tartar).
Yeast	Gluten flour, egg, baking powder.
Non-yeast breads	Essene bread, flat bread, quick bread.
Ground beef	Ground skinless turkey or chicken and tofu -- all good for lasagna, spaghetti, chili, casseroles.
Rice or potatoes	Millet, buckwheat, wild rice, quinoa, Bulgar, Kasha.
Hot dog and sausage	Turkey or chicken sausages, soy sausage.
Pan frying	Pan broiling, baking, or roasting.
Beef stock	Vegetable stock from carrots, onions, leeks, or celery.
Iceberg lettuce	Spinach, chard, chicory, collards, romaine, mustard, curly endive, kale, escarole.

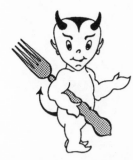

Keeping Food Fresh and Safe

We wanted to give you just a few general tips on how to keep everything in your refrigerator recognizable, as well as preserve nutrients and prevent bacteria growth.

You should always cook frozen food from the frozen state or thaw it in the refrigerator -- not at room temperature.

Freezing merely slows down the growth of bacteria; it does not destroy bacteria. Check our chart for how long to keep foods frozen.

Chicken should be thawed quickly in a microwave or submerged in cold water in order to prevent bacterial growth.

Never forget to wash poultry, fish, pork, etc.; even vegetables and fruits may contain a worm that carries a disease.

All utensils should be washed after cutting to prevent cross-contamination.

Don't eat eggs that are cracked or have not been refrigerated.

Keep your eggs in the carton and refrigerated, not in the egg holder -- as you open and close the door the egg changes temperature.

When you reheat foods, heat them all the way through to at least 165°F.

Veal, beef, and lamb should be heated to 150°F, poultry and pork to 160°F.

Pork should be cooked well -- it may contain larvae and can cause trichinosis, a life-threatening disease.

Acidic foods such as tomatoes or fruit juices shouldn't be stored in cans after opening. It can cause the lead from the can to bleed into the food.

Always check expiration dates on all foods -- give your foods a good looking over -- trust your sense of smell.

If you're at a restaurant and something doesn't look or smell right -- don't eat it.

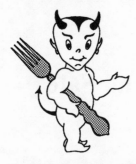

Complementary Side Dishes

You've just finished your main dish, and...it's a masterpiece! Next, you need to decide what to have as your side dish. You need a side dish that will complement your work of art in color, texture, and taste.

Listed below on the chart are several main dishes. Next to each dish are suggested side dishes and salads. At the bottom of all our recipes are side dishes and salads we have already selected from our chart. If you wish, you can choose another side dish or salad that seems appetizing to you.

Main Dish

Suggested Side Dishes

Beef/Pork/Veal

Bread Stuffing
Sweet and Sour
Brussels Sprouts
Mixed Vegetable Bake
Steamed Asparagus*
Herbed Rice Pilaf
Snap Peas and Pearl
  Onions*
Peas and Mushrooms
  with Almonds*
Scalloped Potatoes
Cabbage Salad
Fresh Pineapple Salad
Oriental Spinach Salad
Green Tomato
  Casserole
Potato Puff
Fruited Rice Ring
Baked German Potato
  Salad

Spinach Artichoke Bake
Red Rice
Three Bean Salad
Onion and Tomato
  Savory
Garlic and Sage
  Noodles
Saffron Rice
Cheese Stuffed Potato
Carrots and Basil*
Cauliflower Salad
Swiss Style Green
  Beans
Spinach Salad with
  Lemon Dressing
Saucy Carrot Salad
Baked Apples
Lasagna Florentine
Green Bean Salad
Spinach Casserole

Lamb

Onion and Tomato
  Savory
Cranberries and Raisins
Cabbage Salad
Carrot and Raisin Salad
Sesame Carrots*
Orange Glazed Sweet
  Potatoes
Cashew Rice
Mandarin Spinach Salad
Sweet and Sour
  Brussels Sprouts
Potato Puffs
Spinach Casserole
Bread Stuffing

Sweet Potatoes
Applesauce
Baked Potato
Beet Salad
Herbed Rice Pilaf
Zucchini Salad
Baked Acorn Squash
Oriental Spinach Salad
Spinach Salad and
  Lemon Dressing
Red Rice
Baked Apples
Fruited Rice Ring
Baked German Potato
  Salad

Chicken

Summer Vegetable
  Pasta
Italian Broccoli
Onion and Tomato
  Savory
Peas and Mushrooms
  with Almonds*
Red Rice
Baked Acorn Squash
Fruited Stuffing
Mandarin Spinach Salad
Fresh Pineapple Salad
Saucy Carrot Salad
Fresh Cantaloupe
Garlic Herb and
  Vegetable Salad

Green Tomato
  Casserole
Oat Pilaf
Steamed Asparagus*
Scalloped Potatoes
Cashew Rice
Mixed Vegetable
  Marinade
Cheese Stuffed Potato
Swiss Style Green
  Beans
Oriental Spinach Salad
Herbed Rice
Fruited Rice Ring
Green Bean Salad
Bread Stuffing

Turkey

Scalloped Potatoes
Steamed Asparagus*
Herbed Rice Pilaf
Snap Peas and Pearl
  Onions*
Peas and Mushrooms
  with Almonds*
Carrots with Basil*
Swiss Style Green
  Beans
Oriental Spinach Salad
Green Tomato
  Casserole
Lasagna Florentine
Potato Puffs
Bread Stuffing

Red Rice
Three Bean Salad
Onion and Tomato
  Savory
Garlic and Sage
  Noodles
Saffron Rice
Cheese Stuffed Potato
Company Green Beans
Fresh Pineapple Salad
Cucumber Salad
Saucy Carrot Salad
Fruited Rice Ring
Fresh Strawberries
Fresh Cantaloupe
Garlic Herb and
  Vegetable Salad

Fish

Red Rice
Mandarin Spinach Salad
Snap Peas and Pearl
  Onions*
Almond Spinach Salad
Zucchini Salad
Oat Pilaf
Mixed Vegetable
  Marinade
Saffron Rice
Oriental Spinach Salad
Garlic Herb and
  Vegetable Salad
Herbed Rice
Fruited Rice Ring

Cucumber Salad
Carrots and Basil*
Steamed Asparagus*
Herbed Rice Pilaf
Cashew Rice
Spinach Salad with
  Lemon Dressing
Green Tomato
  Casserole
Saucy Carrot Salad
Tuna Jambalaya
Lasagna Florentine
Wilted Lettuce Salad
Carrots and Cauliflower
  Salad

See recipes for side dishes and salads in this book.

*Fresh or frozen vegetables are easy to prepare without a written recipe. Just add the suggested flavor or mix of vegetables.

Fruited Stuffing

Serves 4-6

Small pkg. cornmeal dressing **1 cup dried mixed fruit, chopped**	Mix together.
1/4 cup onions, chopped **1/2 cup celery, chopped** **1 Tbsp. vegetable oil**	Sauté.
1/2 cup hot water **1 medium egg or egg substitute**	Whip together. Add to the above ingredients. Spray a baking dish with non-stick cooking spray and spoon in stuffing. Bake uncovered at 350°F for 30 minutes.

Oat Pilaf

Serves 4-6

2 medium eggs or egg substitute	Beat with a fork.
3 cups quick cooking oats	Stir into eggs.
3 Tbsp. vegetable oil or margarine	Melt in deep pan. Add oat mixture. Cook and stir until dry and brown.
14 oz. chicken broth **Pinch of thyme and basil**	Stir into the above ingredients. Cook and stir until the liquid has evaporated.
Parsley	Add for garnish.

Italian Broccoli

Serves 6-8

3 lbs. (2 bunches) broccoli
6 cups boiling water
Pinch salt

Cook broccoli until tender. Drain.

1/2 cup olive oil
1 clove garlic, sliced
1/4 cup lemon juice

Toss with cooked broccoli.

Place in serving bowl.

May be served hot or cold.

Potato Puffs

Serves 4-6

1-1/3 cups potatoes

Mash and set aside.

2 eggs or egg substitute

Beat.
Add to mashed potatoes.

1/2 cup low fat milk
1/2 cup water
2 Tbsp. margarine or vegetable oil
1/4 tsp. salt
1 clove garlic, crushed

Heat in saucepan to boil.
Remove from heat and stir in potato mixture.

Drop by teaspoonfuls on a baking sheet.
Refrigerate 1 hour.
Shape into 2 dozen balls.
Bake at 350°F until golden brown.

This is a great snack food too!

Baked Apples

Serves 4

4 large apples

Core and stand upright in baking dish.

1-1/3 cups granola (recipe on page 192)
1/2 tsp. cinnamon
1/2 tsp. coriander
1/2 cup honey
1 Tbsp. vegetable oil
1/4 cup apple juice
1 Tbsp. orange juice

Mix together.
Pack apples with filling.

Cover and bake at 325°F for 25 minutes; until tender.

Mixed Vegetable Marinade

Serves 6-8

1 lb. broccoli, cut into florets
2 yellow squash, cut into thin strips
1 large head cauliflower, cut into
   florets
2 cups carrots, sliced
1 medium red onion, diced

Toss vegetables in a large bowl.

Dressing

1/2 cup vegetable oil
1/4 cup red wine vinegar
2 tsp. sugar
1 tsp. salt
1 tsp. basil
1 tsp. Dijon mustard
1/2 tsp. pepper
Dash nutmeg
2 cloves garlic, crushed

Combine ingredients in jar and shake.

Toss with vegetables.

Chill 1 hour.

May be kept refrigerated in a closed container for 3-4 days.

Baked Acorn Squash

Serves 6

3 small acorn squash or chayote squash	Cut in half lengthwise. Remove seeds and pulp.
2 Tbsp. margarine or vegetable oil 2 Tbsp. honey Dash ground cinnamon	Mix together. Divide evenly among squash halves.
2 apples, chopped Raisins (optional)	Place squash in baking dish. Add water to the dish and cover. Bake at 375°F for 1 hour.

Cheese Stuffed Potatoes

Serves 2

2 medium potatoes, baked	Cut in half and spoon out center.
4 Tbsp. low fat cottage cheese 4 Tbsp. plain low fat yogurt 4 Tbsp. cheddar cheese, grated 1 tsp. dill weed 4 Tbsp. green onion, chopped	Mix all ingredients and blend with potato. Spoon into potato skins. Bake at 350°F for 15 minutes.
Paprika	Sprinkle over potatoes.

Cashew Rice

Serves 4-5

1 Tbsp. margarine 1/2 cup onion, chopped	Sauté.
1 cup brown rice 1 tsp. turmeric	Add to sauté. Stir 2 minutes.
1 tsp. salt 2 cups water	Bring to boil and add rice mixture. Simmer 45 minutes.
1/2 cup cashews	Stir in cashews once rice is cooked.

Scalloped Potatoes

Serves 4-5

3 potatoes, sliced thin	
1/2 cup mushrooms, sliced 1/2 tsp. salt 2 cups cream of mushroom soup	Mix together.
1 pimento pod, chopped 1 medium onion, chopped	Mix together. Arrange 1/3 potatoes in baking dish. Top with 1/3 of the mushroom and 1/3 of the pimento mixture. Repeat. Bake at 350°F for 1 hour.
Paprika	Sprinkle on potatoes.

Saffron Rice

Serves 4-5

1 cup brown rice 1/4 tsp. saffron, crushed	Boil in 2 cups water until cooked.
1 cup onion, chopped 1 clove garlic, minced Dash basil	Sauté and add to rice when cooked.

Various vegetables can be added if desired, like peas or carrots.

Swiss Style Green Beans

Serves 4-6

1-1/2 lbs. green beans	Steam until tender.
1/3 cup lemon juice 2 cloves garlic, crushed 1/2 cup olive oil 1 tsp. tarragon 1 tsp. dill weed 1/4 tsp. salt 2 tsp. Dijon mustard 2 Tbsp. parsley	Mix together and add to green beans.
1 cup green and red peppers, sliced 1/3 cup walnuts, chopped, or almond slices	Add to bean mixture.
4 oz. low fat Swiss cheese	Cut into strips and place on top of bean mixture.
	Chill for 2 hours.

Herbed Rice Pilaf

Serves 4-5

1 cup brown rice 2 cups water 1/8 tsp. salt	Bring to boil in saucepan. Simmer 40 minutes. Cool.
1 Tbsp. sesame oil 1 clove garlic, minced 1/4 tsp. dill 1/4 tsp. basil 1/2 tsp. oregano	Add to rice when cooled.

Sesame Carrots

Serves 4-5

2 cups carrots, diced 2 tsp. sesame seed oil 1 tsp. salt 2 tsp. soy sauce 1/2 cup orange juice 2 tsp. barley malt	Combine ingredients in saucepan. Bring to boil and simmer 5 minutes.
2 tsp. sesame seeds	Sprinkle over carrots.

Snap Peas and Pearl Onions

Serves 4-5

1 lb. snap peas 20 pearl onions 2 Tbsp. margarine or vegetable oil	Sauté.
1 tsp. mint flakes 1/2 cup water	Add to sauté and bring to a boil. Cover, reduce heat and simmer 10 minutes.
1/4 cup cashews	Add to vegetables.

Herbed Rice

Serves 4

3/4 cup brown rice 1-1/2 cups water Dash salt	Bring to boil. Simmer covered 40 minutes.
1/4 cup almonds, chopped 2 Tbsp. vegetable oil	Sauté.
1/3 cup onion, minced Dash pepper 1/4 tsp. rosemary 1/4 tsp. lemon basil 2/3 cup carrots, cooked and diced	Mix and add to sauté. Add rice.

Tuna Jambalaya

Serves 4-6

1 Tbsp. vegetable oil 1 large green pepper, chopped 1 rib celery, chopped	Sauté in large pan.
16 oz. can tomatoes 14 oz. can beef bouillon 1/2 can water	Add to the sauté. Bring to a boil.
1 cup regular rice, uncooked 2 - 6-1/2 oz. cans of tuna (water packed) 1/2 tsp. salt 1/4 tsp. pepper 1/4 tsp. tabasco (optional)	Add to the above mixture. Simmer until rice is tender and liquid is absorbed.

Small cooked shrimp may be added just before serving.
This also makes a nice main dish served with a green salad and rolls.

Fruited Rice Ring

Serves 6-8

1 Tbsp. vegetable oil 1 medium stalk of celery, diced	Sauté in a large pan.
11 oz. pkg. mixed dried fruit, diced (save some whole fruit for garnish) 1-1/2 cups long grain rice 3 cups water 1 tsp. salt	Add to the above ingredients. Cook until rice is tender and liquid is absorbed. Spray 6 cup ring mold with non-stick cooking spray. Spoon rice mixture in mold. Pack lightly. Cover with foil. Bake at 350°F for 20 minutes. Turn onto serving platter. Garnish with remaining fruit.

Baked German Potato Salad

Serves 8-10

1 Tbsp. vegetable oil 1 cup celery, chopped 1 cup onion, chopped	Sauté.
8 cups potatoes, sliced and cooked	Place in large baking dish sprayed with non-stick cooking spray.
3 Tbsp. flour 1-1/3 cups water 2/3 cup cider vinegar	Mix together. Cook and stir until thickened.
2/3 cup sugar 1 tsp. salt 1/2 tsp. pepper	Stir into above mixture. Add onion and celery mixture.
1/4 cup bacon bits (soybean bits)	Pour over potatoes. Cover and bake at 350°F for 30 minutes.

Red Rice

Serves 4-6

1 Tbsp. vegetable oil 1 cup regular rice 1/2 cup onion, chopped 2 cloves garlic, minced	Brown in a large frying pan.
8 oz. can tomato paste 2 cups water 1 green pepper, chopped 1 tsp. paprika 1 tsp. salt 1/4 tsp. chili powder 1/8 tsp. red pepper 1/8 cup bacon bits (soybean bits)	Add to the above ingredients. Cover and cook until rice is tender and liquid is absorbed.

Spinach Artichoke Bake

Serves 10-12

14 oz. can artichoke hearts, drained	Place on bottom of 3 quart casserole dish sprayed with non-stick cooking spray.
3 - 10 oz. pkgs. frozen chopped spinach	Thaw. Drain well. Layer over artichokes.
8 oz. pkg. low fat cottage cheese 2 Tbsp. light mayonnaise 3 Tbsp. vegetable oil	Beat in mixer until fluffy.
6 Tbsp. low fat milk Dash pepper	Beat into the above mixture. Pour over vegetables.
1/3 cup Parmesan or Romano cheese	Sprinkle over above mixture. Bake uncovered at 375°F for 40 minutes or until lightly browned.

You may put this dish together ahead of time and refrigerate before baking. If chilled, increase the baking time approximately 5 minutes.

Lasagna Florentine

Serves 6-8

1 Tbsp. vegetable oil 3/4 cup onion, chopped 2 cloves garlic, minced	Sauté in a large saucepan.
2 - 26 oz. jars of tomato pasta sauce	Add to the above ingredients. Simmer 15 minutes.
10 oz. pkg. frozen spinach	Thaw and drain well.
15 oz. ricotta cheese 1/2 cup Parmesan cheese 2 eggs or egg substitute 1/4 cup low fat milk	Beat well. Mix well with the spinach.
1 cup mozzarella cheese, shredded 1 lb. lasagna noodles, cooked	Spray a 9 x 15 inch dish with non-stick cooking spray. Spoon in 2 cups tomato sauce. Lay on 1/2 lasagna noodles. Spoon 1/2 of remaining tomato sauce. Pour on all of spinach mixture. Sprinkle on 1/2 of mozzarella cheese. Lay on remaining lasagna noodles. Spoon on remaining tomato sauce. Cover with foil. Bake at 350°F for 45 minutes. Top with remaining mozzarella cheese. Bake uncovered an additional 15 minutes. Let stand 5-10 minutes before serving.

Orange Glazed Sweet Potatoes

Serves 4-6

40 oz. can sweet potatoes drained or 3 large yams, cooked, peeled, and chopped

Put potatoes in baking dish sprayed with non-stick cooking spray.

1/4 cup brown sugar
1/4 cup granulated sugar
1 Tbsp. corn starch
1/8 tsp. salt
1 cup orange juice
1 tsp. orange peel, grated

Mix together.
Cook until thickened.

1 Tbsp. margarine

Add to above mixture.
Pour over potatoes.
Bake in microwave on high 3 minutes or in 350°F oven for 30 minutes.

Spinach Casserole

Serves 4-6

2 cups chopped spinach, cooked and drained

Place in baking dish sprayed with non-stick cooking spray.

1 Tbsp. margarine, melted
1 tsp. tarragon
1/2 tsp. salt
Few drops lemon juice
4 oz. can mushrooms, drained

Mix together.
Spread over spinach.

4 eggs or egg substitute

Beat well.

1/2 cup Parmesan cheese

Mix with eggs.
Pour over above mixture.
Bake at 350°F for 30-40 minutes.

Green Tomato Casserole

Serves 4-6

5-6 medium green tomatoes	Do not peel tomatoes. Slice very thin. Layer 1/3 of tomato slices in a baking dish sprayed with non-stick cooking spray.
1 cup bread crumbs **3 Tbsp. margarine, melted** **3 Tbsp. brown sugar**	Sprinkle 1/3 crumbs over tomatoes. Drip 1 Tbsp. margarine over crumbs. Sprinkle with 1 level Tbsp. sugar. Repeat layers. Bake uncovered at 350°F for 30 minutes.

Summer Vegetable Pasta

Serves 4-6

1/2 cup onion, chopped **1 Tbsp. vegetable oil** **1 clove garlic, minced**	Sauté.
1/4 green pepper, chopped **1/2 zucchini, sliced (optional)**	Add to the sauté and cook about 5 minutes.
2 or 3 fresh tomatoes, peeled and cut into chunks **1 cup fresh mushrooms, sliced**	Add to the above and cook just enough to warm. Toss with cooked spaghetti or pasta of your choice.
Parmesan or Romano cheese, grated	Top vegetables and pasta.

Make this a main dish by adding 1/2 pound cooked crab or shrimp.
Serve with a green salad.

Mixed Vegetable Bake

Serves 6-8

6 cups fresh vegetables (such as cauliflower, broccoli, carrots, onions, turnips, rutabaga, etc.)	Cook vegetables until tender. Drain. Place in 1-1/2 quart baking dish sprayed with non-stick cooking spray.
3/4 cup cold milk 1 Tbsp. corn starch 1/2 tsp. salt 1/8 tsp. pepper	Mix together and cook until thickened.
1 Tbsp. margarine	Add to the above sauce and stir until melted.
3 Tbsp. fresh dill or 1 Tbsp. dried 2 Tbsp. lemon juice 1 Tbsp. parsley, chopped	Stir into the above mixture. Toss with vegetables.
1/2 cup bread crumbs 1/4 cup Parmesan cheese, grated 2 Tbsp. parsley	Mix together. Sprinkle over vegetable mixture.
1 Tbsp. margarine, melted	Bake at 350°F for 20 minutes.

Sweet and Sour Brussels Sprouts

Serves 4-5

1 pkg. brussels sprouts	Cook until tender. Drain.
2 tsp. vegetable oil 1 Tbsp. onion, chopped	Sauté.
1 Tbsp. bacon bits (soybean bits) Dash salt and pepper 1 Tbsp. vinegar 1-1/2 tsp. sugar 1/2 tsp. dry mustard	Mix together. Add to onions. Toss with brussels sprouts. Place in serving dish.

Company Green Beans

Serves 6-8

2 - 10 oz. pkgs. green beans

Cook until tender. Drain.

2 Tbsp. margarine
1 cup onion, minced
2 cloves garlic, minced

Sauté until tender.

1/4 cup parsley
1/4 tsp. dried rosemary
1/2 tsp. dried basil

Add to onion and cook 1 minute.
Stir into green beans.
Pour into a serving dish.

Bread Stuffing

Serves 4-6

4 cups dry bread cubes

1 tsp. salt
1/8 tsp. pepper
1/8 tsp. ginger
3/4 cup poultry seasoning
1 tsp. parsley, chopped
2 Tbsp. margarine, melted
1 egg or egg substitute
1 small onion, chopped fine
1 rib celery, chopped fine
1/2 cup hot water

Mix together.

Stuff turkey.

Don't be afraid to add your own favorite ingredients (mushrooms, oysters, water chestnuts, etc.)

Corn Bread Stuffing

Serves 4-6

8 cups corn bread crumbs

1 tsp. salt	Mix together.
1/8 tsp. pepper	
1/8 tsp. ginger	Stuff turkey.
3/4 cup poultry seasoning	
1 tsp. parsley, chopped	
2 Tbsp. margarine, melted	
1 egg or egg substitute	
1 small onion, chopped fine	
1 rib celery, chopped fine	
1/2 cup hot water	

Garlic Sage Noodles

1 pkg. noodles (or use our recipe on page 169 to make your own)	Cook as directed.
1 Tbsp. margarine or vegetable oil	Stir into noodles.
1/4 tsp. garlic powder	Sprinkle over noodles.
1/4 tsp. sage	Stir and serve.

How Long to Keep?

Butter
Refrigerator 1 to 3-1/2
  months
Freezer 6 to 9 months

Cheese
Refrigerator 2 weeks
Freezer 6 months

Eggs
Refrigerator 1 month

Fresh Fish
Refrigerator 1 day
Freezer 3 to 7 months

Cooked Fish
Refrigerator 3 to 4 days
Freezer 4 months

Raw Meat
Refrigerator 1 to 4 days
Freezer 1 year

Raw Poultry
Refrigerator 1 to 2 days
Freezer 7 months

Cooked Poultry
Refrigerator 3 days
Freezer 1 month

Margarine
Refrigerator 3 to 5 months
Freezer 1 year

Flour
Cabinet 6 to 9 months
Refrigerator 1 year

Milk
Refrigerator 1 to 7 days
Freezer 2 months

Yogurt
Refrigerator 1 to 2 weeks
Freezer 1 to 2 months

Ice Cream
Freezer 2 months

Don't allow foods to stand at room temperature for more than 2 hours after cooking.

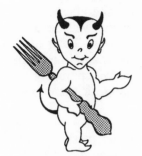

6. Creatively Using Mistakes

Let's be creative and not get in a flap over mistakes. Always think SIMPLICITY.
Don't panic. You can always creatively use your mistakes -- or order pizza. When
we sat down to write this book we had a devil of a time sharing stories about our
mistakes. Even if a meal is a total flop you are still left with a funny story that is
sure to get some laughs for at least a couple of years. Everyone likes a good cooking
disaster story, so I suppose we can share a story or two.

Not all mistakes can be salvaged, but we can learn from them.

Okay. Shortly after Velma was married, she placed some sweet potatoes in the oven
to bake. Suddenly there was an explosion! Cautiously, Velma crept into the kitchen,
not knowing what to expect. She opened the oven and spattered from corner to corner
were sweet potatoes! Velma learned she had to perforate the potatoes with a fork to
let out the steam.

Have you ever had your cream of wheat look like one big lump? If so, next time just
pop it into the blender for a second. This can also be done with sauces that curdle
because they were either cooked too quickly or an acid from an herb or vegetable
caused curdling. Simply blend for a few seconds and the protein will coagulate again
and no one will ever know. If your sauces get too thick, just add a few drops of
water or milk.

What can you do if you add twice as much water to a cake as you're supposed to?
Think simplicity. Take some water out if you still can. If you already stirred up your
batter add a couple tablespoons of cake flour until the batter seems normal. Possibly a
pinch of extra salt or sugar and you're ready to bake.

One weekend many years ago, the family decided to go camping. Velma began to
throw a cake together and realized she had put in twice as much water as needed. She
scooped out some water and finished the cake. To this day the family remembers that
cake as the most moist, rich, delicious chocolate cake they ever had.

Do you tend to eat mostly dark crunchy food? We refer to this as burned. Burning food is one of my talents, so I now use stainless steel pans that reflect some of the heat and prevent excessive burning. Cooking is much easier with a good set of no-stick cookware.

If you still continue to burn food, we have another idea for you that worked for us. Let us explain. On my wedding day, Velma and I forgot that there was another barbecue beef brisket in the oven. After the reception was over and the kitchen cleaned up, we learned that the oven was still on. Inside was a crispy, well done barbecue beef brisket! The meat was wrapped and placed in the freezer. Later in the winter, the meat was thawed and put through the food processor and made into a pot of chili. That was some of the best chili we have ever had and we will probably never be able to reproduce it. You can always make chili, stew, soup, or casseroles from all those dark crispy creations.

Velma found out why a recipe for split pea soup didn't come with her pressure cooker. She had made pea soup in the pressure cooker a number of times. One day it must have been cooking too hard because the pressure regulator blew off and pea soup covered the ceiling. Her first impulse was to grab the cooker and run outdoors with it. Fortunately she didn't because that would have left a trail of soup on the ceiling. The cooker was removed from the heat and allowed to cool. The soup that was left in the pot was just fine and good to eat.

The point is everyone makes mistakes. Don't be too quick to throw out food. Take a good look at it and be creative. Make something good to eat out of your mistake.

Table of Equivalents: Weights and Measures

Moderation

1 dash = 2-4 drops
1 average serving = 4 ounces
1 ounce fluid = 28 grams
4 quarts = 1 gallon
1 quart = 4 cups
1 pint = 2 cups
2 cups = 16 ounces
1 cup = 1/2 pint
1 cup = 8 fluid ounces
1 cup = 16 tablespoons
1/4 cup = 4 tablespoons
2 tablespoons = 1 fluid ounce
4 tablespoons = 2 fluid ounces
1 tablespoon = 1/2 fluid ounce
1 tablespoon = 3 teaspoons

Milliliters
1/2 fluid ounce = 15 milliliters
2 fluid ounces = 60 milliliters
8 fluid ounces = 240 milliliters
16 fluid ounces = 480 milliliters
32 fluid ounces = 960 milliliters or .96
  liters

Flour
Whole wheat 3-1/2 cups unsifted = 1
  pound
White 4 cups sifted = 1 pound
Cake 4-1/2 cups sifted = 1 pound
Pastry 4 cups sifted = 1 pound

1 Cup Fluid
Cooking oil = 200 grams
Milk, soup = 240 grams
Honey, syrup = 325 grams
Water = 220 grams

Cooked Beans
Kidney 1-1/2 cups = 1 pound
Lima 2-1/3 cups = 1 pound
Navy 2-1/3 cups = 1 pound
Soy 2 cups = 1 pound

Notes

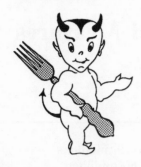

Money Saving and Time Saving Ideas

We want your time spent in the kitchen to be productive and enjoyable. Therefore, we have listed a few money and time saving ideas. Something as simple as keeping things clean and organized in the kitchen can save a lot of time. Preparing meals at home can save money, time, and frustration. Eating fast food is no longer cheap, nor quick. It can take forever to reach the drive through window, only to arrive home and find a chicken sandwich instead of a double cheeseburger!

Save yourself some gas and time. Meals eaten at home usually leave you with leftovers that can be refrigerated or frozen and used for another meal or a snack.

All our recipes utilize common everyday ingredients you may already have in your pantry. We want to save you time, and having to run out for a last minute ingredient makes cooking a hassle and a quick cheeseburger sound good!

It is wise every so often to take an inventory of your pantry, making sure things are stocked and fresh. Also keep old food cleared out of your refrigerator.

Don't go grocery shopping when you are hungry.

Check supermarket ads. Buy large quantities of meats that are on special. Package and freeze it for future use.

Make a list and follow it to control impulse buying. If you have a menu planned for a week, it will help you to shop wisely.

If cookies, crackers, or cereal are stale, simply bake them at 350°F for 2-3 minutes and repackage.

Store whole grain flour in a brown paper bag in the refrigerator or it will get rancid.

Don't store open cans of food in the refrigerator or the lead from the cans will leach into the food.

If bread has gone stale make your own bread crumbs in a food processor or blender. Put them in a tight container and freeze.

Also use stale bread to make croutons.

Stale bread is good to make stuffing and bread pudding.

You can save money when you skin and bone chicken yourself. Use the bones to make chicken stock by simmering in water with a dash of salt and pepper and any desired seasoning. Strain the stock and refrigerate. If you know that the stock will not be used for a couple of days, put it in the freezer.

To bone chicken breasts, start with a sharp knife, slice along the breastbone, pull and scrape the meat away from the bone, ending at the rib edge. On a thigh, slice along each side of the bone, pull the meat and slice away from the ends of the bone. It's easier if the meat is slightly frozen.

Set your oven 25 degrees lower if you are using glass pans; they absorb more heat than other materials.

If you cut vegetables thin or on an angle, it requires less water and cooking time and saves nutrients.

By tearing lettuce instead of cutting it with a knife, you'll slow down the browning due to enzymatic decay.

Save stock from vegetables and meat to make gravy. Refrigerate and let stock solidify -- skim off fat.

Meats have a bright red color due to oxymyoglobin (pigment) and when meat is rewrapped at home it may turn a purple color. Meat is not spoiled, it just lacks oxygen.

Salads with greens may be prepared ahead. Place all ingredients in the bowl, cover, refrigerate. Add dressing just before serving.

Sprinkling lettuce or fruit with lemon juice, orange juice or sugar will keep it fresh longer.

Use your freezer. Most foods can be frozen using a special freezer wrap.

Don't throw out hard cooked eggs that have a green tinge. They are still good. The green color comes from overcooking. To prevent this green tinge, place eggs in water and bring to boil. Remove pan from heat and let eggs stand 10 minutes. Place eggs in cool water.

Foods can spoil quickly. Refrigerate or freeze. Don't let set at room temperature.

Roasting a turkey on a weekend can supply you with countless good tasting meals and a portion can be frozen for later use.

Soups are quick and economical to prepare. Use leftover meat and vegetables and add to stock.

Cheese that has been forgotten in the refrigerator can be trimmed and shredded and wrapped and frozen and used for baking.

Before roasting a turkey breast, slice off a few nice pieces, pound thin or leave as is, separate with wax paper, wrap and freeze for future use.

Make use of a pressure cooker to utilize less tender and less costly cuts of meat. A pressure cooker also saves time. (Recently, after 35 years of use, Velma's pressure cooker fell apart. That's a lot of use!)

When you prepare a roast, plan to have one large enough so you can have hot sandwiches the next day for dinner.

Planning is a big time saver. Think ahead about what you are going to cook. Start first with the foods that will take longer to cook. Set the table, have the coffee maker ready to plug in when you sit down to eat. Working in steps and in an organized order help keep you from getting nervous and excited. As you cook, clean up after yourself. As you clear the table and stack the dishes, put food away at once.

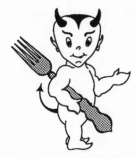

7. Main Dishes

Cooking Trivia: Main Dishes

Fish has little connective tissue, and therefore requires little cooking time. Meats have more connective tissue and require longer cooking time.

The more connective tissue, the less tender the meat.

Salted ham can cause scalloped potatoes to curdle.

Grilled fish is often marinated using oil, lemon, or lime juice to enhance flavor.

Tenderizing meats can be done by scoring across the grain or using a meat tenderizer containing bromelin.

Do not salt meat before cooking; it will delay browning and decrease juiciness.

Round, chuck, and brisket are less tender cuts of meats, and good methods for preparation are to braise, stew, pressure cook, or slow cook.

Rib, loin cuts, T-bone, strip, and porterhouse are tender cuts of meats, and the best methods of cooking are to roast, broil, pan broil, or fry.

Collagen is a connective tissue that disintegrates by moist heat and turns into gelatin. Elastin (gristle) is another connective tissue that doesn't soften by cooking.

Good fish to grill are salmon, lake trout, halibut, shark, and swordfish.

Always thaw fish in the refrigerator, not at room temperature.

Monkfish is known as poor man's lobster.

Cured meat has a permanent pink color due to nitrosomyoglobin.

Research has revealed that the Omega-3 fatty acids found in fatty fish can lower the incidence of heart disease.

Fresh meat has a bright red color due to a pigment called oxymyoglobin and when rewrapped at home will turn purple (myoglobin) from lack of oxygen.

Tuna may be one of six species; albacore, blackfin, bluefin, skipjack, yellowfin, and little tuna.

Cornish hen is a crossbreed of the Plymouth Rock Chicken and Cornish Gamecock. It can be roasted, broiled, or braised.

When fish is done, it flakes when pierced with a fork in its thickest part.

Bake, broil, or roast meats on a rack so the meat remains above the drippings.

Keep your oven closed until the protein in the food has solidified. How do you know when this has happened? Use your sense of smell. When there is an aroma, your proteins are solidifying.

If you want to reduce cholesterol when baking, you can't just cut out all the fat in the recipe. You could use 1 tablespoon of oil for every egg and then some baking powder or baking soda as your leavening agent.

Give dough enough time to rise. If indentation made by inserting two fingers into dough remains, dough rising is complete.

If you are going to make a gelatin salad, don't use fresh pineapple, papaya, or figs. It is the enzyme bromelin that will prevent your gelatin from jelling. The bromelin will keep breaking the protein bonds. That's why pineapple is placed on hams -- it acts as a tenderizer.

If you are going to make an unshortened cake like angel food, do not grease your pan. If you do, your cake will not rise. Many people have made these kinds of mistakes, but usually only once. How do you think we found out about this?

If you're nervous and you keep on rolling your pie crust again and again your crust will not be flaky, but tough. The more you roll, the more gluten you produce, which will toughen your crust.

When making bread with yeast, sugar is important. The yeast eats the sugar and produces carbon dioxide and causes the bread to rise. If you leave out the sugar you'll have a delicious flat chunk of bread.

If you are going to alter ingredients, make subtle changes. It's safer. Maybe we'll develop a kitchen crisis hot line. I'm sure we could all have used the support at some time or another!

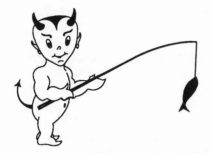

Fish and Seafood

The flavor of fresh fish is outstanding. Most fish can cook in 10 minutes at 350-400°F because it has little connective tissue. You can add or subtract 2 minutes for each 1/4 inch above or below one inch. Fish will flake when done and the translucent appearance of fish becomes opaque.

The best rule of thumb when buying frozen fish is to make sure it is solidly frozen, with no soft spots. The package should be tightly wrapped and no ice crystals should be deposited on the side of the package. The ice crystals hurt cells in the fish's flesh and dry it out.

Quality fish can certainly be found frozen. Quick freezing is the key to preserving fish and seafood. This method uses temperatures of 20 to 40 degrees below zero to freeze. This does not destroy flavor or nutrient content like the Omega 3-Fatty acid. Fish can also be cooked in its frozen state, which keeps fish tender.

If you want to thaw your fish, do so in the refrigerator or place the sealed package under cold running water, not warm. When freezing fish at home, freeze the fish in its original wrapper made with special coated paper designed to retain moisture.

We recommend you eat breaded or battered frozen fish only if there is no other food available. I know they call it fish and that it is hidden somewhere in the thick breading, but..."Where's the fish?" Try grilling fish instead; it gives fish a unique flavor and aroma.

Most people are familiar with cod and ocean perch. But there are so many flavors and textures available in other fish. We have described a few not so common fish you will enjoy trying. Use our charts to help you decide between a lean or fatty fish, and to identify fresh fish.

Selecting Quality Fish

Frozen fish should feel solidly frozen, with no soft spot, which indicates partial thawing.

No ice crystals or frost indicating temperature changes and loose wrapping during storage and transport. Fish will be dry and tasteless.

Fish should have a bright colored flesh, look firm, and rather glossy if it was Quick Frozen.

Freezer burn may appear as white or yellow cloudy looking patches. Totally ruined.

How to Test Your Fish

1. Fish that is <u>properly cooked</u> will have an opaque look, and will have a milky white juice. Fish will flake easily in the thickest part when tested with a fork.

2. Fish that is <u>over cooked</u> will also have an opaque look but there are no juices. It will be dry and not flake but break into small pieces.

3. Fish that is <u>under cooked</u> has a translucent look, and the juices are watery and clear. The flesh is very firm and won't flake easily.

Fat Choices

Lean fish: atlantic pollack, bass, bay and sea scallops, halibut, flounder, haddock, orange roughy, perch, red snapper, shrimp, and sole.

Fatter fish: albacore, bluefish, catfish, herring, lake and rainbow trout, mackerel, salmon, shad, shark, smelt, swordfish, tuna, and whitefish.

Fatter fish are great for grilling.

Not So Common Fish

Bluefish is a delicious fish to broil or grill. It is an oily fish and tastes great with lemon and onion.

Monkfish is known as poor man's lobster. It is good tasting and can be baked, broiled or poached.

Baby coho salmon are milder tasting than regular salmon steaks. They are smaller and are a cross-breed between salmon and trout. Try baking, broiling, pan frying, steaming, or poaching.

Mahi-mahi is a type of dolphin, but is not a member of the porpoise family. Its white meat is popular in Hawaiian cuisine. It has a sweet taste and can be baked, broiled, pan fried, etc.

Salmon Steaks
with Rosemary Mustard

Serves 4

1 lb. fresh or frozen salmon steaks

1 tsp. powdered rosemary
1 small clove garlic, crushed
1/4 cup Dijon mustard
2 Tbsp. vegetable oil

Combine to make a basting sauce. Brush steaks.

Broil 4-6 minutes for each 1/2 inch of thickness. Baste occasionally with remaining sauce. Fish will be flaky when done.

Suggested Side Dishes

Carrots with Basil
Brown Rice

Fillet of Sole with Mint

Serves 4

1 lb. fresh or frozen fish fillets

2 Tbsp. onion, chopped
1 Tbsp. fresh mint, finely chopped
1 Tbsp. lime juice
1 clove garlic, minced
Dash pepper
Dash salt

Combine and place in bowl for basting sauce.

Bake at 400°F for 20 minutes. Baste fish occasionally with sauce.

Suggested Side Dishes

Red Rice
Snap Peas and Pearl Onions

Mackerel Parmesan

Serves 4

1 lb. fresh or frozen mackerel

1/4 cup sesame seed oil
1/4 cup lemon juice
1 Tbsp. dry basil

Combine and pour over fish.
Marinate 1 hour.

1/2 cup Parmesan cheese, grated
1/4 tsp. garlic salt

Combine and coat fish with mixture.

Bake at 400°F for 15 minutes or until flaky.

Suggested Side Dishes

Zucchini Scramble or
Swiss Style Green Beans

Swordfish and Apples

Serves 4

1-1/2 lbs. fresh or frozen swordfish
 steaks

2 Tbsp. margarine or vegetable oil
4 Tbsp. brown sugar or rice syrup
2 large apples, sliced or diced
1/2 tsp. nutmeg

Heat ingredients in frying pan. When margarine is melted add swordfish.
Cover and simmer 10-15 minutes.

Suggested Side Dishes

Oat Pilaf with Almond Spinach Salad

Seafood Lasagna

Serves 6-8

8 lasagna noodles

Item #1. Cook until tender; drain.

1 cup onion or green onions
1 Tbsp. vegetable oil

Sauté.

1-1/2 cups low fat cottage cheese
1 egg or egg substitute
2 tsp. basil
Dash pepper

Item #2. Mix in a blender. Stir in sautéed onions.

1 can cream of mushroom soup
1 can cream of celery soup
1/3 cup low fat milk
1/3 cup white wine

Item #3. Mix together.

1 lb. uncooked shrimp (fresh or frozen)
8 oz. crab meat (can or imitation)

Item #4.

1 cup low fat mozzarella cheese, shredded
1/2 cup Parmesan cheese

Item #5.

Layer ingredients as listed #1, #2, #3, #4, and #5 in large loaf pan sprayed with non-stick cooking spray. Should make 2 layers.

Bake at 350°F for 45 minutes.

1/2 cup low fat cheddar cheese

Remove from oven. Top with cheddar cheese. Let stand 10 minutes. Cut into squares and serve.

If you like a sharp flavor - substitute the cream of celery soup with a can of nacho cheese flavor soup.

Suggested Side Dish

Almond Spinach Salad

Scallops with Ginger

Serves 4

1 lb. scallops, cleaned

3 Tbsp. margarine
1 tsp. ginger root, grated
3/4 cup carrots, shredded
1/2 cup green onions
2 Tbsp. lemon juice

Combine all ingredients in heated skillet and add scallops.

Cook 3 minutes.

Carrots should be crispy and bright colored.

Suggested Side Dishes

Spinach Pasta with
Fruited Rice Ring

Shrimp with Broccoli

Serves 4

12 oz. shrimp, cleaned

4 Tbsp. olive oil
1 clove garlic, minced
Dash basil
Dash oregano
3 Tbsp. lemon juice
3 Tbsp. Parmesan cheese

Combine all ingredients in heated skillet.
Add shrimp.
Cook until shrimp turns pink; about 6 minutes.

Suggested Side Dishes

Cherry Tomato Halves with
Cooked Broccoli

Down Home Fish Stew

Serves 6

3-1/2 cups fish stock or vegetable broth

**1 lb. fish fillets, cut into bite size
   pieces**

1 large jar northern beans, drained

1/2 cup onion, chopped
1/2 cup celery, chopped
3 Tbsp. margarine
1 small head cabbage, chopped
3 Tbsp. parsley, chopped
1 Tbsp. pimento, chopped
Dash pepper
Dash oregano

Combine all ingredients in saucepan
except fish and let simmer, covered for
30 minutes. Stir occasionally.

Add fish and simmer another 5 minutes
until fish flakes.

Suggested Side Dishes

Mandarin Spinach Salad with
Rosemary Whole Wheat Bread

Tuna or Salmon Loaf

Serves 4-6

**2 - 9-1/4 oz. cans tuna or salmon,
   packed in water**
1 medium egg or egg substitute
1/2 cup low fat milk
2 cups bread crumbs
2 Tbsp. green onions, chopped
1/4 tsp. oregano
1/4 tsp. thyme

Mix ingredients together.

Place mixture in loaf pan. Bake
uncovered at 350°F for 40 minutes.

Suggested Side Dishes

Swiss Style Green Beans or
Peas and Carrots

Fruited Stuffed Sole

Serves 4

4 medium sole fillets

1/4 cup brown rice, cooked 1/3 cup raisins and apples, chopped 2 Tbsp. green onions, chopped 1 Tbsp. celery, chopped 2 tsp. orange peel, shredded 2 Tbsp. orange juice Dash salt Dash parsley 1 Tbsp. margarine or vegetable oil	Combine all ingredients in a saucepan and cover. Simmer 15 minutes. Spoon stuffing along the length of each fillet. Roll fillets like a jelly role. Place stuffed rolls in baking dish. Bake uncovered at 350°F for 15-20 minutes.
2 Tbsp. slivered almonds	Sprinkle over baked fish.

Suggested Side Dishes

Orange Slices
Snap Peas and Pearl Onions

Skillet Sautéed Shark

Serves 4

4 medium shark steaks or other fish steak	Place in heated skillet.
4 Tbsp. margarine or vegetable oil 1/4 cup green peppers 1/4 cup onions 2 Tbsp. lemon juice 1/2 cup mushrooms 1-1/2 Tbsp. Dijon mustard	Heat all ingredients in skillet, basting sauce over steaks. Keep turning steaks and cook until fish flakes with fork. Spoon remaining sauce over steaks.

Suggested Side Dishes

Mixed Vegetable Marinade with
Cashew Rice

Flounder with Lemon Sauce

Serves 4

4 medium flounder fillets

Dash pepper
Dash paprika
Dash tarragon

Sprinkle on fillets.
Bake at 400°F for 6 minutes for each
1/2 inch of thickness.

Lemon Sauce Recipe on page 144

Suggested Side Dishes

Cauliflower Salad with
Wild Rice

Breaded Pike Parmesan

Serves 4

4 medium pike fillets

1 cup herb seasoned stuffing croutons,
crushed
1/3 cup Parmesan cheese
2 Tbsp. green onions, chopped
Dash paprika
Dash dill

Mix ingredients in a plastic bag. Toss
each fillet in bag to coat.

Place breaded fillets on baking dish.

Bake at 400°F. Allow 6 minutes for
each 1/2 inch of thickness.

Suggested Side Dishes

Garlic Herb and Vegetable Salad
Brown Rice

Salmon with Seafood Sauce

Serves 4

4 medium salmon steaks

Dash dill
2 Tbsp. olive oil
2 Tbsp. lemon juice

Mix ingredients and brush over salmon.

Bake at 400°F for 6 minutes for each 1/2 inch of thickness.

Seafood Sauce Recipe on page 142

Spoon sauce over fish and sprinkle with parsley.

Suggested Side Dishes

Baked Potato
Carrots with Basil

Broiled Swordfish
with Toasted Almonds

Serves 4

4 medium swordfish steaks

2 Tbsp. lemon juice
2 Tbsp. sesame seed oil
1 tsp. oregano
1/4 cup almonds, finely chopped

Mix together and brush generously over swordfish.

Broil 6 minutes for each 1/2 inch of thickness. Brush fish occasionally with marinade.

Suggested Side Dishes

Hot Fettucini
Carrot and Raisin Salad

Shrimp and Chicken Toss

Serves 4-6

1 whole chicken breast	Skin and bone chicken. Cut into 1/2-inch thick strips.
1/2 lb. medium to large shrimp	Shell and devein shrimp.
2 Tbsp. dry sherry **1 Tbsp. cornstarch** **1 tsp. ginger root, grated or 1/4 tsp. ground ginger** **1/4 tsp. salt**	Toss with shrimp and chicken. In hot oil, stir fry about 2 minutes until chicken is tender and shrimp is pink.
2 Tbsp. vegetable oil **1 lb. mushrooms** **3 Tbsp. soy or tamari sauce**	Cook to boiling over high heat in a 2 quart saucepan. Stir. Reduce heat, cover and simmer 5 minutes.
12 oz. pkg. fettuccine	Cook and drain. Place on a large platter.
1/2 lb. fresh spinach	Wash, drain, and coarsely slice. Place on fettucine in a mound. Add chicken shrimp mixture on top of spinach. Spoon mushroom sauce over the above.
1/2 red pepper, cut into strips	Garnish.

Suggested Side Dish

Sesame Carrots

Simple Baked Fish Fillets

Serves 4-6

4 Tbsp. vegetable oil
2 Tbsp. lemon juice
Salt
Pepper

Mix together.

4 large fish fillets (cod, haddock, sole, or whatever you choose)

Dip fish in oil and lemon.

1/2 cup bread crumbs

Coat fish.

Place in a baking pan sprayed with non-stick cooking spray.

Bake at 500°F for 10-12 minutes.

For smaller batches reduce oil and lemon mixture.

Suggested Side Dishes

Garlic and Sage Noodles
Cabbage Salad

Shrimp Scampi

Serves 4-6

4 Tbsp. margarine	Melt in 9 x 13 inch baking pan under broiler.
2 tsp. garlic, crushed	Mix well.
3 Tbsp. parsley, chopped	Add to the margarine.
2 Tbsp. lemon juice	
1/4 tsp. salt	
1/2 cup dry white wine	
1/2 tsp. dry mustard	
1 lb. medium to large shrimp	Shell and devein. Add to the above ingredients.
	Broil 5 minutes. Stir. Broil another 5 minutes.

Wine may be substituted with chicken broth.

Suggested Side Dishes

Mixed Vegetable Marinade and
Red Rice

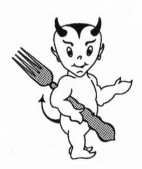

Often you can find shrimp at a good price in pound bags, shelled, deveined, frozen. Thaw in the refrigerator or under cold running water, rinse, and drain.

Steamed Mussels

Serves 4

1 lb. bag mussels	Wash under running water. Remove beards.
1/2 cup onion 2 Tbsp. margarine 1 cup white wine 1/2 cup parsley	Mix together. Place in a large pot. Cover and simmer just until mussels open. Remove mussels to a large bowl. Strain broth through cheesecloth into another pan to remove sand.
1/2 cup low fat milk	Add to broth. Cook until reduced in volume.

Wine may be substituted with chicken broth.

Suggested Side Dishes

Spaghetti or Pasta of your choice
Spinach Artichoke Bake

Fish Rolls with Corn Bread Stuffing

Serves 6

6 fish fillets (sole or whitefish)	Rinse fish in ice water with a dash of salt and lemon added. Drain well on paper towel.
1-1/2 cups packaged corn bread stuffing **1 egg or egg substitute** **1/4 cup hot water** **1 Tbsp. onion, chopped**	Mix together.
Dash salt **Dash pepper** **Dash basil** **Dash thyme** **Dash garlic powder**	Lay fillets out flat. Sprinkle with salt, pepper, basil, thyme, and garlic powder. Place 1 Tbsp. stuffing on each fillet. Roll and secure with a toothpick. Lay rolls seam side down in a baking pan spayed with non-stick cooking spray.
1 tsp. lemon juice **2 tsp. vegetable oil**	Whisk together. Brush on fish. Bake at 450°F about 15 minutes. Fish should be flaky. Be careful not to overcook fish. It gets tough, dry, and loses its flavor.

Suggested Side Dish

Cucumber Salad

Sauce with tiny shrimp is good served on top of fish rolls.

Fish Marinade

Serves 4

2 large fish fillets (any kind desired) (approximately 2 lbs.)

Rinse in ice water with a dash of salt and lemon.
Drain well on paper towel.

Low fat bottled Italian dressing

Just cover bottom of a shallow baking dish with some dressing.
Lay fish in dish.
Spoon more dressing over fish.
Marinate, covered in the refrigerator 30 minutes or longer.

Let as much dressing drain off fish as possible.
Place in a baking pan sprayed with non-stick cooking spray.

Bake at 450°F for 12-15 minutes.

Try this with Saffron or Seafood Sauce from our Sauce Chapter.

Suggested Side Dishes

Saffron Rice with
Oriental Spinach Salad

Cajun Type Red Snapper

Serves 4-6

1 Tbsp. paprika
1-1/2 tsp. salt
1 tsp. onion powder
1 tsp. garlic powder
1/2 tsp. red pepper
1/2 tsp. black pepper
1/2 tsp. thyme
1/2 tsp. oregano

Mix together well.

2 Tbsp. margarine, melted
4 red snapper fillets 1/2- to 3/4-inch
   thick (other firm fillets can be used)

Brush fillets with margarine.

Dip fillets in seasoning.

2 Tbsp. vegetable oil

Heat 1 Tbsp. oil in frying pan until hot.
Cook fillets 2-3 minutes.
Add rest of oil.
Turn fillets and cook another 2-3
minutes.

Suggested Side Dishes

Corn Muffins with
Swiss Style Green Beans

Imitation Crab Alfredo

Serves 4-6

2 Tbsp. margarine
1/4 cup Parmesan cheese
1/4 cup Romano cheese
1/2 cup low fat milk
Dash salt
Dash pepper

Mix together in saucepan.
Heat just enough to mix well.
Set aside.

1 Tbsp. margarine
1 clove garlic, minced
1 lb. imitation crab pieces

Place in large frying pan.
Heat through.

1/4 cup dry white wine
1 Tbsp. lemon juice

Add to above.
Simmer about 2 minutes.
Add all ingredients to milk mixture.
Simmer 2 minutes.

Fettucine

Cook enough for 6 people.
Drain well.
Toss with crab mixture.

2 Tbsp. parsley, finely chopped

Top pasta and crab mixture.

Suggested Side Dish

Spinach Salad with Lemon Dressing

Shrimp Fettucine

Serves 4

1/3 cup olive oil
1 lb. medium shrimp, uncooked, peeled, and deveined
1/2 cup fresh basil, chopped
2 Tbsp. green onions, finely chopped
Dash pepper
Dash paprika
1 Tbsp. Parmesan cheese

Place in large skillet.
Cook over medium heat until shrimp turns pink.

5 medium tomatoes, chopped
1/4 cup pitted black olives, sliced

Add to above ingredients.
Heat through.

1 lb. fettucine, fully cooked

Pour shrimp mixture over fettucine and serve.

Suggested Side Dishes

Herbed Rice
Steamed Asparagus

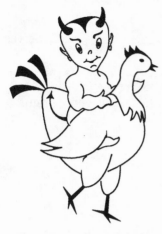

Meats and Poultry

Most of the fat in our diet is hidden fat. After reading this section and preparing several of our recipes, finding hidden fat will not be a mystery. Meats are an excellent source of protein, vitamins, and minerals. It is not necessary to eat large portions of meat to get enough protein. The portion size of meat recommended is a 3 ounce serving of cooked lean meat, fish, or poultry.

By preparing your own meals, you'll not only save money but reduce your fat intake considerably. The meals you eat in restaurants may contain far more fat than you suspect.

The term meats applies to beef, veal, pork, and lamb. If you have any questions, don't hesitate to ask your butcher. It is a misconception to think the fat in meat is what gives it flavor. It's not true. It's the quality of the meat and how it is prepared. An extra lean piece of beef can have more flavor than one marbled with fat.

We have designed several charts that will help you make better choices. Check our chart and select a lean steak not heavily marbled. Good quality lean beef is a consistent bright, light to deep red color. All meats should feel firm and dry, not soft and moist. Choose lean meats for grinding with no visible fat.

If you're buying veal it should be light pink, and there is less fat in younger animals. When buying ham, the butt end of a ham is leaner than the shank end, and the center ham slice has a lot of fat marbling. Lean boiled ham or sliced turkey is a great choice for sandwich meats.

The best method for cooking pork would be roasting or broiling because it is high in saturated fat. Pork needs to be cooked well and the internal temperature of 150°F is necessary to kill trichinae. It is a good idea when preparing stew, soup, or gravy made from meats, to chill and then skim off fat that rises to the top.

Meats...Becoming Food Wise

Nutritional Tips

Trim meat of all visible fat

Beef
Eat lean or extra lean cuts: sirloin, top and bottom round, tenderloin, rump, flank, London broil, brisket (trimmed)

Lamb
Leg or loin chops

Pork
Lean loin, well trimmed ham steak, Canadian bacon

Moderation in serving sizes: 3 ounce cut to 1/2-inch

Salting before cooking will reduce juiciness and delay browning

Have your butcher grind round steak instead of hamburger

To keep lean meats tender: Braise, stew, pressure cook, cook in liquid or use low heat and long cooking time

USDA Grading System

Prime: Contains the most fat

Choice: Lean, less tender than prime

Select: Contains least fat

Lean: Must have a fat contents of 10% or less

Extra Lean: Must have a fat content of 5% or less

The American Heart Association recommends that Americans eat no more than 6 ounces of fish, lean or extra lean meat, or skinless poultry a day.

Cooking Terms

Bake: To cook by dry oven heat.

Braise: To brown in water or broth.

Baste: To moisten food while it is cooking or roasting by spooning or brushing a mixture over it.

Blanch: To make skin of fruit or nuts easy to remove by steeping them in boiling water a few minutes.

Julienne: Food cut in long thin strips.

Knead: Using hands to stretch, press and fold a mixture and make it smooth.

Marinate: To soak foods in a mixture usually containing oil with vinegar, lemon juice and/or wine, for flavor and tenderizer.

Mince: To put through a press or mincer or to chop finely.

Parboil: To boil until partly cooked.

Pare: To remove the skin of fruit or vegetable with a knife.

Pan Fry: To cook in a skillet on top of the stove with a small amount of oil.

Poach: To simmer in liquid below boiling point.

Roast: To cook uncovered without water in oven.

Sauté: To brown quickly in oil, broth, etc. on top of stove.

Sear: To brown the surface of meat at high temperature in heated skillet either in oven or on top of stove to seal in juices.

Stew: To cook uncovered on a rack placed under or over direct heat.

Stock: The liquid in which fish, meat, or vegetables have been cooked.

Beef Stew with Oat Bran Crust

Serves 4-6

2 lbs. lean beef chunks 1 Tbsp. vegetable oil	Brown meat in oil in Dutch oven or large frying pan.
1 large onion	Remove meat from pan. Sauté onion. Replace meat.
13-14 oz. beef broth 2 Tbsp. Worcestershire sauce 1/4 tsp. pepper 1 tsp. salt	Add to the meat and onion. Simmer until tender.
4 (about 2 lbs.) sweet potatoes, peeled and cubed 4 (about 1 lb.) parsnips, peeled and sliced	Add to meat mixture and cook covered until tender.
1 Tbsp. flour 2 Tbsp. cold water	Mix together and add to the above ingredients.

Oat Bran Crust

1 cup flour 1/4 cup oat bran 1/4 cup parsley 1 tsp. baking powder 1/2 tsp. salt 6 Tbsp. margarine	Blend together.
3-4 Tbsp. milk	Add to the above ingredients 1 Tbsp. at a time. Refrigerate 15-20 minutes. Roll out and place over stew. Bake at 425°F for 15 minutes.

Suggested Side Dishes

Onion and Tomato Savory
Spinach Salad with Lemon Dressing

Italian Beef Rolls

Serves 6-8

2-1/2 to 3 lbs. boneless bottom round steak

Trim all fat from the roast.
Make thin slices; about 3 by 5 inches.
Meat slices easier if slightly frozen.

Garlic powder
Salt
Pepper

Sprinkle over meat slices.

1/4 lb. hard salami, sliced very thin
1/4 lb. mozzarella cheese, sliced very thin

Lay a slice of cheese and salami on each slice of beef.
Roll and secure with toothpick.

2-3 Tbsp. vegetable oil

Brown rolls in oil in a Dutch oven.

Spaghetti sauce

Nearly cover rolls with sauce.

Bake covered at 325°F for 2 hours or until well done.

Serve with your favorite pasta.

Suggested Side Dishes

Italian Broccoli or
Oriental Spinach Salad

Rouladen

Serves 6-8

2-3 lbs. boneless round beef roast

Trim fat from meat.
Slice thin, about 3 by 5 inches.
Meat slices easier if slightly frozen.

Prepared mustard
1 large onion
6 dill pickles
Dash salt
Dash pepper
Dash garlic powder

Spread each meat slice with mustard.
Sprinkle with salt, pepper, and garlic
powder.
Lay thin slice of onion and pickle on
each.
Roll and secure with a toothpick.

2 Tbsp. vegetable oil

Brown rolls in oil in a Dutch oven or
deep baking dish.
Nearly cover with water.

Bake covered at 325°F for 2 hours or
until tender.

3/4 cup water
3 Tbsp. flour

Whisk together.

1 small can mushrooms or 1/2 cup
fresh mushrooms

Remove meat rolls from the broth.
Thicken broth with flour mixture.
Add mushrooms.
Pour gravy in large bowl.
Add rolls and serve.

Suggested Side Dishes

Three Bean Salad with Potato Puffs
Garlic and Sage Noodles

Special Beef Stew

Serves 6-8

4 lbs. lean beef 1/2 cup flour 4 Tbsp. vegetable oil	Cut meat in 1/2-inch slices. Dredge with flour. Brown in 2 Tbsp. oil in frying pan. Remove meat to Dutch oven.
2 lbs. large onions, thick sliced 6 cloves garlic, minced	Sauté onions and garlic in remaining oil. Add to meat.
3 Tbsp. brown sugar 1/4 cup red wine vinegar 1/2 cup parsley, chopped 2 small bay leaves 1 Tbsp. salt 2 tsp. thyme leaves Freshly ground pepper 2 - 10-1/2 oz. cans beef broth 2 - 12 oz. bottles of beer	Mix ingredients in same pan used for browning meat and preparing sauté to make sauce. Add to meat. Bake covered at 325°F for 2 hours or until very tender. Remove from oven.

Dumplings

2 cups flour 4 tsp. baking powder 1/2 tsp. salt 1 scant cup low fat milk	Mix dumplings and drop onto stew. Cover and return to oven for 10-15 minutes.

This is a great party dish.
Can be put together the day before and refrigerated until baking time.

Suggested Side Dishes

Green Bean Salad
Saffron Rice

Beef with Pea Pods

Serves 4-6

1 lb. flank or sirloin beef (can also use chicken or turkey)	Slice into strips.
1 green onion	Slice onion into chunks.
1 Tbsp. soy sauce **1 Tbsp. vermouth** **2 Tbsp. corn starch**	Mix together. Stir into meat and onions. Marinate 1/2 hour or longer.
1 Tbsp. oil	Heat oil. Stir fry above ingredients until brown.
1 pkg. frozen, thawed or 1/4 lb. fresh pea pods	Stir fry in a separate pan about 5 minutes in 1 Tbsp. hot oil.
	Stir meat and pea pods together.

Suggested Side Dish

Herbed Rice Pilaf

Whole Beef Tenderloin

Serves 4

1 to 1-1/2 lbs. beef tenderloin

Place on broiling pan.
Broil 15 minutes per pound for rare, 20 minutes for medium rare, 30 minutes for well done.

Place meat on platter.
Slice.
Spoon hollandaise sauce over meat. (See our recipe on page 143.)

Suggested Side Dish

Sautéed Matchstick Thin Carrots and Rutabaga
Wilted Lettuce Salad

Sukiyaki

Serves 6

2 lbs. lean beef
2 Tbsp. vegetable oil

Slice beef into strips.
Sauté in oil.

2 medium onions, cut into chunks
2 bunches green onions, sliced
5 cups celery, sliced diagonally

Add onions and celery to meat.
Cook and stir until tender.

1/2 lb. fresh mushrooms, sliced
2 - 5 oz. cans water chestnuts, sliced

Add to the above ingredients.
Heat through.

2 cans beef broth
4 Tbsp. corn starch
3/4 cup soy sauce
1/2 cup sherry

Mix well.
Add to the above mixture.
Cook and stir until thick.

1 pkg. fresh spinach

Tear into pieces and stir into Sukiyaki.

Suggested Side Dish

Brown Rice

Barbecue Beef Brisket

Serves 8-10

6 lbs. beef brisket

Trim off fat.

1 can beef broth

Mix together.

1/4 cup lemon juice
1 small bottle soy sauce

Place meat in deep dish.

1 Tbsp. liquid smoke

Pour sauce over meat.

Dash garlic powder

Cover and let marinate overnight, turning

1 cup barbecue sauce

meat every few hours.

Bake tightly covered in sauce at 300°F
for 3 hours.

1 cup barbecue sauce

Pour 1 cup barbecue sauce over the meat
and cook uncovered at 350°F for another
hour.

Place on platter.
Slice across grain.
Spoon a little broth over meat before
serving.

This is a great buffet party dish.

Suggested Side Dishes

German Potato Salad
Green Tomato Casserole
Cauliflower Salad

London Broil

Serves 4-6

2 lbs. flank steak

Trim excess fat.

1-1/2 Tbsp. safflower oil
1 tsp. lemon juice
1/8 tsp. pepper
1/8 tsp. salt
1 clove garlic, minced
2 tsp. parsley, chopped

Combine and brush over steaks.

1 cup white mushrooms, sliced

Sauté in remaining oil mixture.
Place steaks on oiled broiler pan.
Brush one side with seasoned oil mixture and broil for 5 minutes.
Turn steak and brush with seasoned oil mixture and broil an additional 5 minutes.

Slice steak very thin on a diagonal.

Serve topped with mushrooms.

Suggested Side Dishes

Snap Peas and Pearl Onions
Cheese Stuffed Potatoes

Easy 5 Hour Stew

Serves 4-6

2 lbs. lean beef, cut into cubes
6 carrots, cut into 2 inch pieces
4 medium potatoes, quartered
5 celery stalks, sliced diagonally
1 green pepper, sliced
1 large onion, chopped in large pieces

Place all ingredients in Dutch oven.

1/4 cup tapioca
2 tsp. salt
1 tsp. sugar
1 large can stewed tomatoes

Add to the above ingredients and stir well.

Bake covered at 250°F for 5 hours.

Don't peek!

1/4 cup shredded cabbage may
  also be added

Good busy day dinner. If you have a timer on your oven, your dinner is ready when you walk into the house.

Suggested Side Dish

Sunflower Seed Bread

Braised Veal Chops with Fennel

Serves 4

4 veal chops 1-1/2 inch thick

In skillet, heat 2 Tbsp. vegetable oil over medium heat. Brown chops on both sides.

2 Tbsp. dry white wine
1/4 tsp. fennel seed, crushed
1/8 tsp. pepper
1/4 tsp. sugar
1/2 tsp. salt
1/4 cup onion, chopped
3/4 cup carrots
8 oz. tomatoes
1/3 cup green peppers, chopped

Add all ingredients to veal. Reduce heat and cover. Cook for 1 hour or until chops are tender.

Suggested Side Dishes

Baked Potatoes
Cranberries

Sweet and Sour Pork

Serves 4-6

6 medium lean pork cutlets

1 tsp. ginger	Mix and coat cutlets.
1 tsp. salt	
1/2 tsp. pepper	
1 tsp. paprika	
1/4 cup flour	

1 Tbsp. sesame seed oil or vegetable oil   Brown cutlets in large frying pan.

1 cup pineapple juice   Mix and add to cutlets.

2 Tbsp. vinegar

3 Tbsp. brown sugar or honey   Cover and cook over low heat 40 minutes.

Suggested Side Dish

Corn with Basil and Carrots
Fruited Rice Ring

Honey Baked Pork

Serves 6-8

3 lbs. lean boneless pork loin roast   Place in a deep dish.

1 cup ginger ale   Mix together and pour over the roast.
1/2 cup honey   Cover
1/2 cup Dijon mustard
1/4 cup vegetable oil   Marinate in refrigerator at least 1 hour.
**2 Tbsp. onion powder or chopped
  onion**   Remove meat from marinade.
1-1/2 tsp. rosemary   Place in baking pan.
1/2 tsp. salt   Bake covered at 350°F for 30 minutes
1 tsp. garlic powder   per pound. While baking, baste with
1/4 tsp. pepper   marinade.

Simmer leftover marinade 5 minutes.
Serve with the roast.

Suggested Side Dishes

Sweet and Sour Brussels Sprouts
Saffron Rice

Barbecued Pork Roast

Serves 6-8

4-6 lbs. lean boneless pork roast

Place in deep dish.

1 can beef broth
1/4 cup lemon juice
1 small bottle soy sauce
1 Tbsp. liquid smoke
Dash garlic powder
1 cup barbecue sauce

Combine.
Pour over roast.
Marinate covered in the refrigerator
overnight.

Place in baking pan.
Nearly cover with marinade.
Cover tightly.
Bake at 300°F for 3 hours.

1 cup barbecue sauce

Remove from oven.
Pour 1 cup barbecue sauce over meat.

Bake uncovered 1 hour.
Slice.
Spoon marinade over meat to serve.

Suggested Side Dishes

Fruited Rice Ring
Oriental Spinach Salad

Great Buffet Party Dish!

Tasty Pork Pie

Serves 4-6

2 Tbsp. vegetable oil
2 lbs. very lean pork

Brown pork in deep frying pan with 1/2 of the oil. Remove meat from pan.

1-1/2 cups onion, chopped
1 clove garlic, minced

Sauté in remaining oil.
Return meat to pan.

1 cup carrots, sliced
2 Tbsp. flour
1 tsp. salt
1/4 tsp. thyme
1/4 tsp. cloves
1/8 tsp. pepper
1 bay leaf
1 beef bouillon cube
1 cup water
1/2 cup dry white wine

Mix together.
Pour over the meat.

Simmer covered until tender. About 45 minutes.

1/4 cup bacon bits
1/4 cup parsley

Stir into the above ingredients.
Cook 15 minutes.

Spray a 10 inch pie dish with non-stick cooking spray.
Roll out pie crust and place in dish.
Pour meat mixture into the crust.
Top with another crust.
Make small slits in top to let out steam.

Bake at 400°F for 15 minutes. Reduce heat to 350°F and bake for another 20 minutes.

Suggested Side Dishes

Cabbage Salad or
Spinach Salad with Lemon Dressing

Orange Marmalade Glazed Baked Ham

Serves 10-12

8 lb. boneless ham

Place fat side down on rack in open roasting pan.
Insert meat thermometer in center.
Bake uncovered at 325°F until internal temperature is 140°F, about 3 hours.
Remove thermometer.

1/2 cup orange marmalade
1/2 cup honey
2 tsp. dry mustard
1 tsp. basil

Spread 1/2 glaze mixture on ham and bake 10 minutes.
Spread remaining glaze on ham and bake an additional 10 minutes.

Good for buffet party dish or family get together.

Suggested Side Dish

Cheese Stuffed Potatoes

Turkish Shish Kabob

Serves 4-6

2-3 lbs. lamb	Cut in 2 inch cubes.
1 large onion, minced **4 onions, cut into wedges** **2 large tomatoes, cut into wedges**	Place in large bowl with lamb.
1/2 tsp. cinnamon **1 Tbsp. salt** **1 tsp. pepper** **1/2 cup vinegar** **1/2 cup vegetable oil** **1 tsp. paprika**	Whisk together. Pour over above ingredients. Marinate in refrigerator for 3 hours. String on skewers, alternating vegetables and meat. Place on broiling pan. Place under the broiler or on the grill 8-10 minutes, turn and broil another 8-10 minutes. Heat marinade and serve over shish kabob.

You may also want to add 1 green pepper, cut into squares and 1/4 cup fresh mushrooms.

Suggested Side Dishes

Herbed Rice Pilaf

Greek Lamb Shanks

Serves 4

1 lb. lamb shanks Flour Salt Pepper	Flour, salt, and pepper lamb. Place in 4-5 quart Dutch oven.
1 large onion, thinly sliced 1 medium green pepper, cut into strips	Place over lamb.
8 oz. can tomato sauce 1 clove garlic, minced 1/2 cup dry white wine or chicken broth 1/2 tsp. salt 1/2 tsp. oregano 1/4 tsp. sugar 1/4 tsp. cinnamon 1/4 tsp. rosemary	Stir well and pour over above ingredients. Bake covered 325°F for 2-1/2 to 3 hours.
1 tsp. lemon juice 1 Tbsp. parsley 2 cups frozen, fresh, or canned green beans	Add to Dutch oven 1/2 hour before cooking time is complete.

Suggested Side Dishes

Herbed Rice
Sesame Carrots

Roast Leg of Lamb

Serves 6-8

5-8 lbs. leg of lamb
2 fresh cloves garlic
Salt
Pepper

Make several incisions in lamb with a
sharp knife.
Insert a thin slice of garlic in each
incision.
Salt and pepper.
Place in a roasting pan.

Roast at 325°F for 30 minutes per
pound.

To avoid fatty gravy, remove lamb to a
platter, cover and keep warm.

Put drippings in a flat bowl.
Place bowl in freezer 5-10 minutes.
When fat begins to solidify, skim it off
the top.
Pour remaining sauce in a pan and heat.

Gravy

3/4 cup water

Add to hot meat drippings.
Bring to boil.

1/4 cup water
2 Tbsp. flour

Whisk together.
Add to the above.
Cook and stir until thick and smooth.

Salt and Pepper to taste
1 tsp. parsley
Pinch thyme

Stir in the above and serve.

If you prefer not to serve gravy with
your leg of lamb, the gravy can be made
later and used to make lamb curry.

Suggested Side Dishes

Baked Potatoes
Spinach Casserole
Carrot and Raisin Salad

Lamb Curry

Serves 4-6

1-1/2 Tbsp. vegetable oil **2 Tbsp. onion, chopped**	Sauté onion in oil.
1 Tbsp. flour **1-2 tsp. curry powder**	Stir into sauté and cook for a few minutes without browning.
2 cups chicken bouillon	Stir bouillon into the above ingredients. Cook until sauce is thick and smooth.
2 cups leftover cooked lamb, cubed	Add lamb and heat through. Serve with boiled rice.

Raisins, chopped apples, and chopped peanuts are good served on the curry. Or you may use prepared chutney.

Suggested Side Dishes

Oriental Spinach Salad
Saffron Rice

Easy Moussaka

Serves 4-6

1 fairly large eggplant

Peel eggplant if desired.
Slice lengthwise 3/8 inch thick.
Blanch in boiling, salted water about 3
minutes, until barely tender.

Or eggplant slices may be cooked
slightly in the microwave.
Place in one layer on paper towel.
Cook on high 1 to 1-1/2 minutes.

1 Tbsp. vegetable oil
1 cup onion, minced

Sauté.

1 lb. ground lamb

Add to onions and brown.

1-2 cloves garlic, minced
1/4 tsp. rosemary
1/4 tsp. thyme
Salt
Pepper

Blend into the above ingredients.

1 cup tomato sauce (bottled spaghetti
 sauce)

1/2 cup mozzarella cheese, shredded
1/3 cup Parmesan cheese

1/2 cup low fat cottage cheese
1 egg or egg substitute
1/4 cup low fat milk

Mix together in blender or mixer.

In a 9 x 12 baking dish sprayed with
non-stick cooking spray, lay half of
eggplant on the bottom.
Place 1/2 lamb mixture on eggplant then
1/2 sauce.
Pour on all of the cottage cheese
mixture.
Sprinkle on half of mozzarella and
Parmesan cheese.
Repeat to form another layer.
Cover dish with foil.
Bake at 375°F for 25 minutes.

Suggested Side Dishes

Spinach Salad with Lemon Dressing or Beet Salad

Lamb Turnovers

Serves 4-6

1 lb. ground lamb
1/2 Tbsp. vegetable oil

Put in large frying pan and brown.

2 green onions, sliced or 1/4 cup
  cooking onion, chopped

Add to lamb.
Cook until tender.

1/2 cup carrot, shredded
1/4 cup raisins
1 tsp. curry powder
1/2 tsp. salt
1/2 tsp. cumin
1/4 tsp. pepper
7-1/2 oz. can tomatoes, cut up
1 medium green pepper, chopped

Stir into the above.
Cover and cook 10 minutes.

If still liquid after 10 minutes, cook uncovered for 3-4 minutes, until liquid is
absorbed.
Remove from heat and cool.

Pie crust recipes pages 171-173

Roll approximately 8-10 inch rounds.
Place in pie tin or on a cookie sheet.
Spoon lamb mixture onto half of the
crust. Fold crust over filling, making a
half round and seal the edges. Make 2
or 3 slits in crust to let out steam.
Bake at 400°F for 30 minutes.

Can be wrapped and frozen for future
use. (If frozen, bake at 400°F for 40
minutes.)

Fruit Sauce (to serve over turnover)

3/4 cup frozen orange juice, diluted
1/4 cup water
1 Tbsp. corn starch

Mix together.
Cook and stir until thickened.

1 Tbsp. raisins or currents

Add to the above mixture.

Sauce can be made in the microwave.
Cook on high, stirring every 40-60
seconds, until thickened.

Suggested Side Dishes

Steamed Asparagus with Applesauce

Turkey Breakfast Sausage

Serves 4

1 lb. ground turkey
1/4 tsp. salt
1/4 tsp. sage
1-1/2 Tbsp. parsley flakes
1/2 tsp. marjoram leaves
1/4 tsp. nutmeg
1/4 tsp. pepper
2 Tbsp. low fat milk

Mix ingredients in medium bowl.

Form into 8 patties and brown in large skillet over medium heat for 15 minutes.

You can freeze what you don't use.

Suggested Side Dishes

Orange Slices with
Whole Wheat Toast

Marinated Honey
and Herb Turkey Breast

Serves 6-8

Place in plastic bag.

3 lbs. turkey breast

1 cup ginger ale
1/2 cup honey
1/2 cup Dijon mustard
1/4 cup vegetable oil
2 Tbsp. onion powder
1-1/2 tsp. rosemary
1/2 tsp. salt
1 tsp. garlic powder
1/4 tsp. black pepper

Mix together very well the remaining ingredients. Pour over the meat. Marinate in the refrigerator 1 hour.

Remove meat from marinade. Put in baking dish and bake at 350°F for 1-1/2 hours (30 minutes per pound).

Simmer leftover marinade and serve with the meat.

Suggested Side Dishes

Oat Pilaf and Mandarin Spinach Salad

Turkey Turnovers

Serves 4-5

1 lb. ground turkey
1 Tbsp. vegetable oil

2 green onions, chopped or 1/4 cup
cooking onion, chopped

7 oz. can tomatoes, cut up
1 medium green pepper, chopped
1/2 cup carrots, shredded
1/4 cup raisins
1 tsp. curry powder
1/2 tsp. salt
1/2 tsp. cumin
1/4 tsp. pepper

Place turkey and oil in a large frying pan and brown.

Add to the above and cook until tender.

Stir in the remaining ingredients. Cover and cook 10 minutes. Cook uncovered another 3-4 minutes if still liquid. Cool.

Roll out pie crust, place in a greased pie tin or on a cookie sheet, spoon filling on half of crust. Fold crust over filling, making a half round and pinch edges together. Prick top of crust to let out the steam.

2 pies will fit into one pie tin. Makes 4-5 good sized pies.

Bake at 400°F for 30 minutes.
If frozen bake at 400°F for 40 minutes.

Suggested Side Dish

Spinach Salad with Lemon Dressing

Turkey Cutlet Parmesan

Serves 4

4 turkey cutlets

1/4 cup unbleached white flour **1/4 tsp. pepper** **2 Tbsp. Parmesan cheese**	Mix together and coat turkey cutlets.
1/3 cup mushrooms, sliced **2 Tbsp. margarine or vegetable oil** **1 small onion**	Sauté and place cutlets in skillet. Brown on both sides. Cover and cook over medium heat for 20 minutes.

Suggested Side Dishes

Saffron Rice with
Cucumber Salad

Turkey Stroganoff

Serves 4-6

1 lb. ground turkey **1 medium onion, chopped** **1 cup mushrooms** **1/4 tsp. nutmeg** **Dash pepper**	Sauté in large skillet over medium heat for 15 minutes.
1-1/2 cups low fat cottage cheese **1 Tbsp. lemon juice** **1/4 tsp. parsley**	Purée in blender. Add to sauté and heat through.
8 oz. pkg. fettucine, cooked	Spoon turkey mixture over fettucine.

Suggested Side Dish

Spinach Almond Salad

Turkey Meatballs

Serves 4-6

1 lb. ground turkey
1 medium onions, chopped
1 cup bread crumbs
1 tsp. salt
1/4 tsp. pepper
1/4 tsp. dill
1 medium egg or egg substitute
2 Tbsp. low fat milk

Mix together in large bowl.
Shape into 1 inch meatballs.
Cook in skillet over medium heat, using non-stick cooking spray, until brown.
Remove meatballs from skillet.

8 oz. vegetable broth (can use vegetable bouillon cubes)
1/4 cup unbleached white flour

Stir together.
Add to juice in skillet and heat.
Stir until gravy thickens.
Return meatballs and warm.

Suggested Side Dishes

Garlic and Sage Noodles or
Cashew Rice

Turkey Casserole

Serves 4

3 cups leftover turkey, cubed
4 oz. can mushrooms
1 can water chestnuts, sliced
1/4 cup blanched almonds
3/4 cup celery, sliced
1 cup light cream of chicken soup
3/4 cup light salad dressing
1/4 cup sherry

Mix together.
Place in a 3 quart baking dish that has been sprayed with non-stick cooking spray.

1 can chow mein noodles

Top casserole with noodles.

Bake at 325°F for 35 minutes.

Suggested Side Dishes

Spinach Salad with Lemon Dressing

Turkey and Egg Deluxe

Serves 6-8

16 slices white bread
Butter flavored cooking spray

Remove crusts from bread.
Spray 9 x 13 inch pan or dish with cooking spray.
Lay 8 slices of bread in the pan and spray them.

1 lb. cooked turkey, sliced
4-1/2 oz. can mushroom slices, drained
or 1/4 lb. fresh mushrooms, sliced
1/4 cup green pepper, sliced
1/2 lb. farmer's cheese, grated or
reduced fat Swiss cheese, grated

Layer half of these ingredients on the bread, in order listed.

Spread remaining 8 slices of bread with margarine and lay on the above.

Layer on remaining ingredients.

2 cups low fat milk
4 eggs or egg substitute, beaten
1 Tbsp. Worcestershire sauce
Dash salt
Dash pepper
Dash thyme
Dash basil
Dash garlic powder

Mix together.
Pour over above ingredients.
Cover and refrigerate overnight.

Bake uncovered at 325°F for 1 hour until custard is set and cheese is brown.

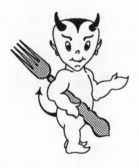

This is a nice dish for company breakfast, brunch, or lunch; especially since it is put together the day before.

Suggested Side Dishes

Fresh Strawberries or
Fresh Cantaloupe

Roast Turkey Breast

Serves 6-8

Whole or half turkey breast

Place breast in a large baking dish that has been sprayed with non-stick cooking spray.

1/4 tsp. salt
1/8 tsp. pepper
Dash each basil, thyme, savory, and garlic powder

Sprinkle on turkey.

1/4 cup dry white wine or water

Add to the above.
Bake covered at 325°F for 2-1/2 to 3 hours.
Add more liquid as needed.

Suggested Side Dishes

Saffron Rice
Green Tomato Casserole

Turkey Cutlet Mozzarella

Serves 4-6

4-6 turkey cutlets

Pound thin.

1/4 cup low fat milk
1/2 cup bread crumbs

Dip cutlets in milk then coat with bread crumbs.

Dash each salt, pepper, basil, thyme, and garlic powder

Sprinkle on the cutlets.

1 Tbsp. vegetable oil

Brown cutlets on both sides in a frying pan.

Tomato, sliced thin
Low fat mozzarella cheese, sliced thin

Lay on each cutlet.
Cover pan and simmer 10 minutes.

Suggested Side Dishes

Summer Vegetable Pasta
Zucchini Scramble

Turkey Breast Florentine

Serves 6-8

1 to 3 lb. turkey breast	Bone turkey and pound to 11 x 8 inch piece.
1 Tbsp. vegetable oil **1/2 cup onion, chopped** **1/4 cup bacon bits**	Sauté onions. Add bacon bits to sauté.
3 Tbsp. flour **1/2 tsp. tarragon**	Mix with the sauté.
1-1/2 cups low fat milk	Add to the above mixture. Cook and stir until thickened.
10 oz. pkg. frozen spinach **2-1/2 oz. can mushrooms**	Cook the spinach and drain. Add spinach and mushroom to 1/2 of the sauce. Chill remaining sauce. Place turkey skin side down. Top with spinach mixture. Roll and tie with string. Place on rack in a baking pan. Cover loosely with foil and bake at 350°F for 1-1/2 hours. Uncover and remove string and bake an additional 30 minutes. Slice and serve.
1/4 cup low fat cheddar cheese, **shredded**	Add to chilled sauce. Heat and serve over turkey.

Suggested Side Dishes

Fruited Rice Ring
Baked or Boiled Potatoes
Company Green Beans

Roast Turkey

Turkey	Defrost in the refrigerator. About 24 hours for each 6 lbs. of weight. Wash well with cold water inside and out. Scrape inside. Drain.
Stuffing (see our recipe on page 35)	Stuff when ready to put turkey in the oven. DO NOT stuff before it's time to cook the turkey. It can be a good place for bacteria to grow.
	Place turkey in roasting pan breast side up. Spray with cooking spray.
Salt **Pepper** **Paprika** **Garlic Powder**	Sprinkle over the turkey.
1/4 cup water	Pour in the roaster. Cover with foil. Add more water if needed.
	Bake 30 minutes per pound for a 6-12 pound turkey. (A 16-20 pound turkey takes approximately 5 to 6-1/2 hours.)
	Turkey should feel tender when tested with a fork.
	If using a meat thermometer, it should register 185° inserted in the thickest part of the drumstick (be certain not to touch the bone).

The size of your turkey depends on how much you like turkey. We think the larger, the better. Leftovers are great! There is a lot to be creative with.

Suggested Side Dishes

Sweet Potatoes with Swiss Style Green Beans

Turkey Cordon Bleu

Serves 4-6

6 slices uncooked turkey breast	Pound into 1/8 inch thick cutlets.
1 tsp. paprika **1 Tbsp. flour**	Sprinkle on turkey.
1 Tbsp. vegetable oil	Lightly brown turkey in frying pan.
6 slices Canadian bacon **6 slices low fat Swiss cheese**	Lay turkey on paper towel. Put a slice of bacon and cheese on each one. Fold in half and secure with a toothpick.
1 Tbsp. flour **1/4 tsp. salt** **1/8 tsp. pepper** **3/4 cup water** **1 cube chicken bouillon**	Stir into frying pan drippings. Stir and cook to thicken.
1/2 cup low fat milk	Add to the above. Cook until smooth. Return cutlets to sauce. Simmer 10 minutes.
2 medium carrots, cut matchstick thin **1 medium zucchini, cut matchstick thin** **Dash salt**	Place in another frying pan that has been sprayed with non-stick cooking spray. Cover and simmer until tender.
1/2 cup low fat milk	Add to vegetables and heat through.
6 oz. vermicelli	Cook as directed on package. Drain.
	Toss with vegetable mixture.
	Place cutlets on a platter and pour vegetable sauce over them.
	Place vermicelli in a large serving bowl.

Suggested Side Dishes

Cucumber Salad
Snap Peas and Mushrooms

Chicken Teriyaki

Serves 4

4 chicken breasts, skinned and boned

1/4 cup tamari
1-1/2 Tbsp. honey
2 Tbsp. lemon juice
1/4 cup water
2 cloves garlic, crushed

Combine ingredients and pour over chicken breasts (saving some for sauce). Marinate overnight in covered bowl.

1 Tbsp. flour
2 Tbsp. cold water

To thicken marinade for sauce, mix flour and water slowly and gradually add to hot marinade.

Bake chicken uncovered at 350°F for 40 minutes, basting every 15 minutes.

Suggested Side Dishes

Herbed Rice Pilaf with Mandarin Oranges and Mint Leaf Salad

Grilled Chicken Thigh Cutlets

Serves 4-6

6 chicken thighs

Bone and pound with meat mallet.

1/4 cup low fat Italian dressing

Spoon half of dressing into a flat dish. Lay chicken in dish and spoon remaining dressing over chicken.

Cover and refrigerate 30 minutes or longer.

Remove chicken from dish and let as much dressing drip off as possible.

Place on a hot grill. Cover and cook 5 minutes on each side. (May also be broiled 5 minutes on each side.)

Suggested Side Dishes

Fruited Rice Ring with Oriental Spinach Salad

Saffron Chicken

Serves 4

4 medium chicken breasts, skinned and boned

Combine and brush over chicken breasts.

4 tsp. olive oil
1/2 tsp. saffron powder
1 tsp. thyme

Bake at 325°F for 60 minutes. Baste chicken every 20 minutes.

Suggested Side Dishes

Cheese Stuffed Potatoes with
Fresh Pineapple Salad

Marinated Honey
and Herb Chicken

Serves 6

3 lbs. chicken breasts

1 cup ginger ale
1/2 cup honey
1/2 cup Dijon mustard
1/4 cup oil
2 Tbsp. onion powder
1-1/2 tsp. rosemary
1/2 tsp. salt
1 tsp. garlic powder
1/4 tsp. black pepper

Mix together with meat. Place in plastic bag. Marinate in refrigerator 1 hour.

Remove meat from marinade. Place in baking dish and bake at 350°F for 30 minutes per pound. Simmer leftover marinade and serve with meat.

Suggested Side Dishes

Oat Pilaf with
Italian Broccoli

Creamy Almond Chicken

Serves 4

4 medium chicken breast halves	Skin, bone and season with pepper.
2/3 cup sliced almonds **1 Tbsp. margarine or vegetable oil**	Sauté.
3 Tbsp. margarine or vegetable oil **Dash salt** **Dash pepper** **1 cup low fat milk** **3 Tbsp. orange marmalade** **1/8 tsp. red pepper**	Combine and heat ingredients slowly.
1/4 tsp. flour **2 Tbsp. cold water**	Mix together slowly and gradually add to heated ingredients to create a creamy low fat sauce. Baste each piece of chicken with sauce. Bake at 325°F for approximately 30 minutes. Pour remaining sauce over baked chicken and sprinkle with sliced almonds.

Suggested Side Dishes

Green Tomato Casserole

Chicken Kiev

Serves 4-6

1/2 cup margarine, softened 1 Tbsp. parsley 1 Tbsp. chives 1 Tbsp. onion, minced 1/4 tsp. salt 1/8 tsp. pepper	Mix together in a small bowl. Chill.
3 whole chicken breasts	Skin and bone chicken. Cut into 6 pieces and pound thin with a meat mallet. Divide margarine into 6 parts and place one on each piece of chicken. Roll and secure with a toothpick.
1/4 cup flour	Dredge with flour.
1 egg or egg substitute Dash salt and pepper 1 Tbsp. cold water	Whisk together. Dip rolls in egg mixture.
1/2 cup bread crumbs	Coat chicken rolls with crumbs.
2 Tbsp. vegetable oil	Brown rolls in frying pan.

Mushroom Sauce

2 Tbsp margarine, softened 1/2 cup onion, minced	Sauté in frying pan used for the chicken rolls.
1 cup low fat milk 1 Tbsp. flour 2 Tbsp. lemon juice Dash salt and pepper	Whisk together and simmer about 5 minutes to thicken.
1 lb. mushrooms, sliced or 2 - 5 oz. cans, drained	Add to above and cook 1 minute. Place chicken rolls on a platter. Spoon some sauce over them.
8 oz. noodles (or other pasta of your choice)	Cook as directed. Toss with remaining sauce.

Suggested Side Dishes

Mixed Vegetable Marinade

Chicken Nuggets

Serves 6-8

3 whole chicken breasts

Bone and cut into cubes.

1 egg or egg substitute, slightly beaten
1/2 cup water
1/2 tsp. salt
2 tsp. sesame seeds
1/2 cup flour

Mix thoroughly.
Dip chicken in batter to coat.

Vegetable oil

Cook chicken in just enough oil to brown and cook.

Dipping Sauce

1 cup catsup
1/2 tsp. dry mustard
1 Tbsp. brown sugar
2 tsp. vinegar
2 Tbsp. vegetable oil

Whisk together.
Cook 5 minutes.
Serve with nuggets.

Suggested Side Dishes

Mixed Vegetable Bake
Scalloped Potatoes
Baked Potatoes
Mandarin Spinach Salad

Easy Pan Baked Chicken

Serves 4-6

6 pieces chicken (any)

Remove skin.
Brown chicken over low heat in a frying pan that has been sprayed with non-stick cooking spray.

1/4 tsp thyme
1/4 tsp. basil
1/4 tsp. salt
1/4 tsp. garlic powder
1/4 tsp. pepper
1/4 tsp. paprika

Sprinkle over chicken.

2 Tbsp. water

Add to chicken.
Cover and cook over low heat until tender, turning occasionally, approximately 30-45 minutes.
Add more water if necessary.

Suggested Side Dishes

Bread Stuffing
Cranberries and Raisins
Cabbage Salad
Italian Broccoli

Stir Fried Chicken

Serves 4-6

3 medium chicken breasts, boned and skinned

Cut into strips. Sauté in non-stick pan until nearly done.

1 Tbsp. peanut oil
1 small head cauliflower
3 stalks celery, cut into 1-1/2 inch diagonal pieces
15 medium mushrooms, sliced
6-1/2 oz. canned water chestnuts, drained
1 medium red pepper, cut into strips
1 medium green pepper, cut into strips
1 cup bean sprouts

In a wok, heat peanut oil. Add all vegetables and stir fry 5 minutes. Add chicken and sprouts. Stir fry 2 minutes.

1/4 cup tamari
2-1/2 Tbsp. rice vinegar

Combine and pour over chicken vegetable mixture.

Suggested Side Dishes

Spinach Salad with Lemon Dressing and Cashew Rice

Papaya Stuffed Cornish Hens

Serves 4

2 medium cornish hens

Remove and discard giblets from hens.
Rinse under cold water and pat dry.
Remove skin and trim fat.
Sprinkle with paprika and pepper.

2 large papayas, cut into bite size pieces
2-1/2 cups plain stuffing mix
2 cups water
1 tsp. sage
1 tsp. basil
1-1/2 Tbsp. fresh ginger root, peeled and chopped
1 medium clove garlic, chopped
2 Tbsp. honey

Mix together.
Spoon into cavity of hens.

Bake at 450°F for 60 minutes.
Place leftover stuffing in baking dish and bake until top becomes brown.

Suggested Side Dish

Swiss Style Green Beans or Lasagna Florentine

Chicken Oriental

Serves 6-8

3 whole chicken breasts — Bone and cut into pieces.

1 Tbsp. corn starch
3 Tbsp. soy sauce
2 Tbsp. dry sherry
1 tsp. sugar
1 tsp. ground ginger
1/4 tsp. red pepper

Mix in a bowl.
Add chicken pieces.
Let stand in refrigerator.

1/2 cup vegetable oil
3 medium zucchini, sliced
1 lb. small mushrooms, sliced
6 oz. pkg. frozen pea pods, thawed

Place in a hot frying pan.
Cook vegetables until tender.
Remove from pan.

Add chicken mixture to the pan.
Stir fry to cook; about 10 minutes.

Return vegetables to the pan and heat through.

Place on serving platter.

Suggested Side Dishes

Herbed Rice Pilaf
Fresh Pineapple Salad

Dijon Chicken Breast

Serves 4-6

3/4 cup water
3/4 cup dry white wine
1 small onion, sliced
3 Tbsp. lemon juice
3/4 tsp. chicken bouillon
12 whole peppercorns
8 sprigs fresh thyme or 1 tsp. dry
  thyme

Mix together in a frying pan.
Cover and simmer 5 minutes.

4 whole chicken breasts, boned

Add to the above pan.
Cover and simmer 15 minutes.
Remove chicken and keep warm.
Strain the broth.

1 Tbsp. honey
2 tsp. Dijon mustard

Add to the broth and cook 10 minutes.

2 Tbsp. water
2 tsp. flour

Mix together and add to the above.
Cook to thicken.

1-1/2 cups fresh mushrooms, sliced

Stir into sauce and cook 2-3 minutes.

Place chicken on serving platter.
Pour gravy over chicken to serve.

Suggested Side Dishes

Baked Acorn Squash
Oat Pilaf
Cashew Rice
Spinach Artichoke Bake

Chicken Stew
and Biscuits

Serves 4

6 pieces chicken, legs and thighs	Remove skin.
1 Tbsp. vegetable oil	Place in a large pan and brown.
1/2 cup water	Add to the pan and simmer chicken 30 minutes.
2 onions, cut in chunks	Add to the chicken and cook 15 minutes
2 ribs celery, sliced	or until the vegetables are tender.
4 carrots, sliced	
1/2 cup frozen peas	Remove chicken from pan and take the meat off the bones.
1/4 tsp. thyme	Add to the above ingredients.
1/4 tsp. basil	Mix well.
1/4 tsp. parsley	
1/4 tsp. garlic powder	
1/4 tsp. pepper	
1 chicken bouillon cube	
1-1/2 cups cold water	Whisk together.
5 Tbsp. flour	Add to the above and cook until thickened.
	Return chicken to pan and heat through.
1 Tbsp. parsley	Stir into chicken mixture.
	Serve over baking powder biscuits.

Suggested Side Dish

Tossed Salad

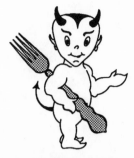

8. Vegetarian Cooking

Vegetarianism is widespread, and was even practiced in ancient Greece and Rome. Vegetarianism takes many forms and there are four types. The total vegetarian, sometimes called vegan, will not eat foods of animal origin, only plant foods.

Through carefully planned food combining, vegans can get the protein, calcium, zinc, iron, and B12 they may lack. Also, vegetarian diets are high in fiber, which tends to bind zinc, making it less available for absorption. A pure vegan will eat only raw plant food, and a lacto-ovo-vegetarian will not eat foods of animal origin, but will eat milk, eggs, and other dairy products.

Lacto-vegetarians eat dairy products, but will not eat eggs. Ovo-vegetarians eat eggs, but will not eat dairy products.

The American Dietetic Association recognizes that well planned vegetarian diets can be nutritionally sound, but growing children, and pregnant and lactating women must take special care to avoid nutritional risk.

We have created several delicious vegetarian recipes that are simple and nourishing. However, throughout our cookbook we have numerous vegetable and fish dishes that could also be enjoyed.

Vegetarian Tostadas

Serves 4-6

16 oz. can refried beans

Heat beans.

6 corn tortillas, baked

8 oz. zucchini slices
2 tomatoes, chopped
1 cup iceberg lettuce, chopped

Combine and toss together.

2 medium avocados
1/2 cup salsa
Dash pepper
1 tsp. lemon juice

Mix together.

Spread beans on tortillas.
Add salsa and avocado mixture.
Top with lettuce mixture.

Gingered Sweet Potatoes

Serves 4-5

4 medium sweet potatoes, scrubbed

Cook until tender.
Peel and purée in blender.

1 Tbsp. margarine
1 Tbsp. honey
1 Tbsp. fresh ginger root, peeled and
   finely chopped
1/4 tsp salt
1/4 cup walnuts and pecans, finely
   chopped

Add to puréed potatoes.

Two ways to prepare:

Place potato mixture in baking dish.
Bake at 350°F for 35 minutes.

or

Using a pastry bag, fill bag with potato
mixture and swirl out onto baking dish
or pan.
Bake at 350°F for 30 minutes.

Tomato and Ricotta Sandwich

Serves 2

4 oz. low fat ricotta cheese
1 large tomato, sliced
1 Tbsp. onion, chopped
1/4 tsp. basil
4 slices rye bread, toasted

Warm in microwave or eat cold.

If desired, sprinkle with sunflower seeds and/or alfalfa sprouts.

Spicy Beans

Serves 4-5

1 cup dry navy beans
1 cup dry pinto beans

Soak and simmer beans as usual. Drain.

1/4 tsp oregano
1/4 tsp. pepper
1/4 tsp. thyme
1 small bay leaf
3 Tbsp. onion, chopped
1/2 cup green and red peppers, diced
1-1/2 tsp. Dijon mustard
4 oz. jar pimentos, diced and drained
1/4 cup cider vinegar
1 Tbsp. olive oil

Add to cooked beans and heat for 15 minutes.

Serve hot or cold.

Acorn Squash with Apple and Onion Stuffing

Serves 4

4 acorn squash halves, with seeds scooped out	Bake until tender.
3 cups tart apples, chopped 1 cup onion, chopped 1/2 tsp. salt 1/2 tsp. thyme 1/4 tsp. pepper	Sauté until tender.
3/4 cup plain bread crumbs 1/4 cup walnuts, chopped 1 egg or egg substitute	Mix together. Add to sauté. Spoon stuffing into cavity of squash. Bake at 375°F for 10 minutes.

Zesty Lentil Salad

Serves 2

1 cup dry lentils 3 cups water	Cook for 30 minutes.
1 bay leaf 1/4 tsp. pepper 1 tsp. thyme 1 tsp. basil 2 Tbsp. olive oil 1/4 cup red wine vinegar 1 small clove garlic, minced 1 small mint leaf	Add to cooked lentils. Let simmer for 10 minutes.
1 cup onion, chopped 1/2 cup carrot, shredded	Add to above mixture. Simmer for 10 minutes.

Vegetarian Pizza

Serves 4

Easy Dough

1 pkg. dry yeast	Knead dough.
1 tsp. sugar	Cover and let rise in warm place for 20
1 cup warm water	minutes.
1 Tbsp. vegetable oil	Roll out dough and fit to pizza pan.
1 tsp. salt	Bake at 350°F for 5 minutes.
3 cups unbleached white flour	Add topping.

Pizza Topping

1 cup crushed pineapple, drained	Place on dough.
1/2 cup fresh basil, chopped	
2 cloves garlic, minced	
6 medium tomatoes, chopped	
1/2 cup mushrooms, sliced	
1/3 cup almonds, sliced	
2 small yellow, red and green bell peppers	
1 Tbsp. oregano	

Spinach Lasagna Roll-Ups

Serves 4

8 lasagna noodles, cooked

10 oz. pkg. leaf spinach, chopped	Combine in large bowl.
15 oz. low fat ricotta cheese	
1/4 cup onion, chopped	
1 Tbsp. parsley	
1 Tbsp. oregano	

16 oz. tomato sauce	Spread ricotta and spinach mixture over length of each noodle.
	Add tomato sauce and roll up noodle.
	Bake at 350°F about 35 minutes.
	Can be frozen and popped in microwave for a quick meal.

Stuffed Mushrooms

1 dozen white button mushrooms,
  cleaned

1/4 cup walnuts, chopped	Sauté 10 minutes.
1/4 cup water chestnuts, chopped	Stuff each mushroom cap.
1/4 cup green onions, chopped	
2 medium cloves garlic, chopped	Place on baking dish and bake at 375°F
2 Tbsp. olive oil	for 8 minutes.
1 Tbsp. teriyaki sauce	
1 Tbsp. parsley, chopped	If desired, sprinkle with shredded
	mozzarella or cheddar cheese and melt.

This makes a great appetizer!

Cold Carrot Soup

Serves 4

15 carrots	Cook in boiling water until tender.
	Purée in blender.
2 cups vegetable broth or vegetable	Add to carrots and purée.
bouillon cubes	
2 cups plain vanilla yogurt	Chill for 30 minutes and serve in soup
1/2 tsp. ground nutmeg	bowls.
1/2 tsp. parsley	Sprinkle with chives.
	Can also be served warm.

Spinach Pesto

Serves 4

10 oz. spinach, chopped	Clean, cook and drain.
3 Tbsp. pesto sauce	Mix together.
1/4 cup plain yogurt	Toss with spinach.
1/4 cup Romano cheese, grated	
Dash pepper	Bite size pieces of baked and seasoned
	tofu can be added if desired.

Vegetable Couscous

Serves 6

1-1/2 cups couscous (semolina)
2 cups water

Bring water to boil.
Simmer 10 minutes.

2 Tbsp. margarine or vegetable oil
1/2 cup green pepper, chopped
1/2 cup red pepper, chopped
3 medium turnips, chopped
1 large zucchini, sliced
1 medium red onion, chopped
1/2 cup peas
1 cup carrots, sliced

Stir fry over medium heat until
vegetables are tender.

1/3 cup walnuts, chopped
1/3 cup raisins
3-1/2 cups tomatoes, chopped

Add to stir fry.
Mix well.

Spoon cooked vegetables over couscous.

Wild Rice with Pecans

Serves 6

1/2 cup wild rice
1/2 cup long grain brown rice
2-1/2 cups water
Dash salt

Bring rice to boil in water and salt.
Reduce heat and simmer 45 minutes.

2 Tbsp. sesame seed oil
1/4 tsp. thyme
1 Tbsp. fresh parsley, chopped
2/3 cup carrots, diced
1/2 cup corn
1/2 cup green peas
1/3 cup onion, chopped
1/3 cup green onions, chopped
1/3 cup zucchini, chopped

Cook until vegetables are tender.

2 Tbsp. pecans, chopped

Add to the above ingredients once
vegetables are cooked.

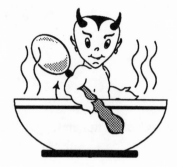

9. Soups, Chowders, and Stews

It's time to put on the soup pot! There's nothing better than a warm bowl of chicken soup when you get struck with the common cold. Those of you who love soups, chowders, and stews, but have yet to make your own, will be surprised at how easy they are to prepare.

Soup is an economical dish, and your leftover meats and vegetables can be used. You can use the tops of celery, or other vegetables that have lost their freshness. Repeated heating of soup is not destructive to its taste, and it can still be enjoyed after several reheatings.

Our recipes include soups, chowders, and stews. Chowder is a thicker creamy dish than soup and usually is made with fish or seafood and sometimes corn or potatoes. Stews and soups consist of meat or various vegetables cooked until tender by slow boiling or simmering. However, stew is served with the sauce produced in cooking. Once you make your own homemade soups you'll never want canned soup again.

Minestrone Soup

Serves 4-6

1 clove garlic, minced 3/4 cup onion, chopped 3 Tbsp. olive oil	Sauté
3/4 cup carrots, diced 3/4 cup celery, minced Dash pepper 1 tsp. oregano 1 tsp. basil	Add to sauté. Cook 8 minutes.
3-1/2 cups water 2 cups tomato purée 3/4 cup green peppers, chopped 1 cup garbanzo beans 1/4 cup parsley	Add to above ingredients and simmer covered 15 minutes.
1/2 cup macaroni noodles	Add noodles and cook an additional 8-10 minutes.

Corn Chowder

Serves 4-6

2 Tbsp. margarine 1 cup onions, chopped 1/2 cup celery, minced	Sauté.
1 sweet red pepper, minced 4 cups (4-5 cobs) frozen corn 1/2 tsp. salt 1 cup stock or water	Add to above ingredients.
1 cup low fat milk	Before adding milk, use your blender to purée about 1/2 the solids in your soup's own liquid. Add milk 10 minutes before serving.

Mushroom Barley Soup

Serves 6

1/2 cup raw pearl barley
6-1/2 cups stock or water
1 tsp. salt
4 Tbsp. tamari
3-4 Tbsp. dry sherry

Cook in soup kettle.

2 Tbsp. margarine or vegetable oil
2 cloves garlic, minced
1 cup onions, chopped
1 lb. mushrooms, sliced
Dash pepper

Sauté.
Add to barley when cooked.

Cream of Celery Soup

Serves 6

4 cups water
4 cups celery, chopped
2 cups potatoes, cut in 1-inch chunks
1 tsp. salt

Bring to boil.
Cook covered until soft.
Purée.

1 clove garlic, chopped
1 cup onion, minced
1 cup celery, minced
1/4 tsp. celery seed
1/4 tsp. salt
3 Tbsp. margarine or vegetable oil

Sauté until tender.
Add to purée.

1 cup low fat milk
1/4 cup plain yogurt
Dash pepper

Add to soup.
Mix well.

Warm soup gently and serve.

Creamy Onion Soup

Serves 4-6

2-1/2 cups low fat milk

Heat very slowly in saucepan.
Remove from heat before boiling.

2-3/4 cups onion, sliced
2 Tbsp. margarine or vegetable oil
1/2 tsp. salt or Worcestershire sauce
1/2 tsp. dry mustard
Dash white pepper
Dash black pepper
Dash nutmeg

Sauté all ingredients.

2 Tbsp. unbleached white flour

Add to sauté.

Add milk.

Stir well.
Cover and let simmer 20 minutes over low heat.

Top with croutons (see page 171).

Bean Soup

Serves 4-6

12 oz. dry mixed beans	Cover with water. Soak for 2 hours and drain.
6 cups water	Place in pot with beans and simmer 2 hours.
1 Tbsp. vegetable oil 1 medium onion, chopped	Sauté. Add to beans.
1/4 cup bacon bits	Add to the above.

1 carrot, sliced
8 oz. tomato juice
1 cup water
1 Tbsp. lemon juice
1 tsp. salt
1/8 tsp. pepper
1/2 tsp. thyme
1/2 tsp. basil
1/2 tsp. tarragon
1 clove garlic, minced or 1/4 tsp.
  garlic powder
1/2 cup cooked chicken pieces
  (optional)
	Add all ingredients to the pot.
	Simmer covered 1/2 to 1 hour.

Essence of Mushroom Soup

Serves 6-8

8 cups water 2 medium onions, chopped 2 lbs. mushrooms, minced 2 tsp. salt 1 Tbsp. fresh lemon juice	Add together in large pot. Bring to boil. Simmer 1-1/4 hours. Strain through a fine sieve lined with cheesecloth.
1/4 cup Madeira wine 1 tsp. salt 1/4 tsp. pepper	Add to above broth. Heat. To serve, garnish with thin slices of mushrooms, scallions or radishes.

Extra Good Chile Con Carne

Serves 4-6

3-1/2 lbs. boneless beef bottom roast or other very lean beef	Trim all fat and cut into chunks.
1 Tbsp. vegetable oil	Brown meat in oil. Remove from pan.
1 Tbsp. vegetable oil 1 large green pepper, chopped 1 medium onion, chopped 1 clove garlic, minced	Sauté.
1 tsp. red pepper 2 Tbsp. chili powder 1-1/4 tsp. cumin 28 oz. can tomatoes 12 oz. can tomato paste 12 oz. bottle beer 2 Tbsp. dark brown sugar 1-1/2 tsp. oregano 1-1/2 tsp. salt	Return meat to pot. Add remaining ingredients. Simmer uncovered until meat is very tender, about 2 hours.
2 - 15 oz. cans red beans	Add to above. Simmer another 15 minutes.

Quick Chicken Soup

Serves 4

1 tsp. vegetable oil 1/4 cup onion, chopped 1/4 cup celery, chopped	Sauté in a saucepan.
3-4 cups chicken stock 1/4 cup cooked chicken pieces 1 Tbsp. chicken bouillon powder	Add to the sauté. Simmer 5-10 minutes.
1/2 cup frozen chopped spinach	Add to above ingredients. Heat and serve.

Danish Sweet Soup

Serves 4-6

1 quart water
1 cup prunes
1 cup raisins
1 cinnamon stick

Place in a 2 quart saucepan.
Simmer about 1 hour.

1 cup tapioca
1/2 cup fruit juice (orange)
1/4 cup sugar

Add to the above.
Simmer until tapioca is clear.

Serve hot or cold.

You may also use packages of mixed dried fruit.

Cucumber Soup

Serves 4

2 cups low fat milk
1/4 cup low fat cottage cheese
2 Tbsp. green onion, chopped
1 tsp. salt

Place in blender.
Blend well.

1-1/2 cups cucumbers, seeded and
   grated

Add to above ingredients.
Chill 2-3 hours.

To serve, garnish with slices of
cucumbers or chives.

Summer Soup
(Gazpacho)

Serves 6-8

1 clove garlic, minced 1 medium onion, chopped 2 cucumbers, chopped 2 large tomatoes, peeled and chopped 1/2 large green pepper, chopped	Place in a large bowl.
2 - 8 oz. cans tomato sauce 2 cans beef bouillon 1/4 cup wine vinegar 1/4 cup vegetable oil 1/4 tsp. tabasco sauce 1 tsp. salt	Add to the vegetable mixture. Stir well. Chill several hours.
1/2 tsp. quick ground black pepper	Add before serving.

This is very good to have on hand.
It may be kept in the refrigerator 4-5 days.

Quick and Easy
Seafood Chowder

Serves 4

1 cup cooked rice 6-1/2 oz. can crab meat 1 small can shrimp 1 can light mushroom soup 2 cups low fat milk 1/2 tsp. salt 1/4 tsp. Worcestershire sauce	Mix together in a saucepan. Heat through. Serve.

Bouillabaisse

Serves 10-12

1 dozen little neck clams 1 dozen medium mussels	Scrub under running water, removing beards.
1 cup water	Place in 8 quart pot. Bring to boil. Add clams and mussels. Cook just until shells open. Remove to a large bowl. Pour broth into a small bowl. Let stand to settle sand. Wipe the large pot.
3 medium leeks, cut into 3/4 inch pieces, or 3 celery ribs 1 clove garlic, minced 2 Tbsp. vegetable oil	Add to the large pot. Sauté until tender.
1 tsp. salt 2 cups water 2 - 14 to 16 oz. cans tomatoes, chopped 3/4 tsp. thyme 1/2 tsp. saffron Broth from mussels and clams, strained if necessary	Add to the above ingredients. Heat to boiling.
2 lbs. boneless cod or scrod, cut into 1-1/2 inch pieces 1 lb. sea scallops, sliced in half 1 lb. large shrimp, cleaned and deveined	Add to above liquid. Reduce heat to medium. Cook 5-10 minutes. Do not overcook or the seafood will become tough. Add clams and mussels. Heat through.
2 Tbsp. parsley	Sprinkle over bouillabaisse. Serve in very large bowls with fresh rolls or garlic bread.

Fish Chowder

Serves 4-6

1 Tbsp. vegetable oil **1/2 cup onion, chopped**	Sauté in a large pan.
1 cup chicken broth **2 cups water** **3 cups potatoes, cut into small chunks** **1/4 tsp. pepper** **1 tsp. salt** **Dash garlic powder** **1/2 tsp. basil** **1/2 tsp. savory**	Add to the above. Cook 5 minutes, until potatoes are tender.
1 lb. cod or haddock	Cut into small pieces. Add to the above. Cook 10 minutes.
2 cups low fat milk **8 soda crackers**	Add to the above mixture. Heat through.
2 Tbsp. liquid margarine **1 Tbsp. flour**	Mix. Add to the above. Cook 2-3 minutes.
1 Tbsp. parsley	Sprinkle into the chowder.

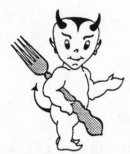

Try one of our bread recipes for an accompaniment.

Danish Clear Soup

Serves 4-6

1-1/2 lbs. lean beef or 3 each chicken legs and thighs, skinned	Place meat in a large pot. Cover with cold water. Bring to a boil. Skim.
1/2 tsp. salt **1/4 tsp. pepper** **1/4 tsp. garlic powder** **1 Tbsp. parsley**	Stir into the above.
2 medium onions, cut into chunks **2 carrots, sliced** **1 stalk celery, sliced**	Add vegetables to the pot. Simmer until tender. Remove meat and vegetables to a serving plate and keep warm. Strain broth through cheesecloth. Return broth to the kettle and heat.

Dumplings

1/2 cup boiling water **1/4 cup margarine**	Mix together. Cool.
1 cup flour **1 egg or egg substitute**	Add to water and margarine. Stir together until smooth. Bring broth to a boil. Drop dumplings in by spoonfuls. Dumplings are done when they rise to the top.

Horseradish Sauce

1 Tbsp. margarine, melted **1 Tbsp. flour**	Stir flour into margarine.
1 cup water	Heat with flour mixture until thickened.
1/4 cup currents **1 tsp. vinegar** **1 tsp. sugar** **2 tsp. horseradish**	Add to the water and flour mixture. After serving the soup, serve the meat and vegetables with the sauce poured over them.

Corn Chowder

Serves 4

1/2 cup onion, chopped
1/2 cup green pepper, chopped
3 Tbsp. margarine or vegetable oil

Cook in a saucepan 5 minutes until tender.

1 tsp. dill weed
1/4 cup unbleached white flour
1 tsp. paprika
1/2 tsp. Worcestershire sauce

Stir into above ingredients.

4 cups low fat milk

Stir into above mixture until thick.

2 - 16 oz. cans whole kernel corn

Do not drain corn.
Add to above mixture.

1 oz. cheddar cheese, shredded

Serve chowder in soup bowls.
Sprinkle with cheese.

Salmon Chowder

Serves 4-6

2 cups fresh or frozen broccoli
1/2 cup onion, chopped
1/2 cup green pepper, chopped
1 Tbsp. margarine or vegetable oil
1/2 cup fresh or frozen corn
1/3 cup celery, chopped

Cook in saucepan until tender.

2-1/2 Tbsp. unbleached white flour
1/4 tsp. basil
1/2 tsp. thyme
3 cups low fat milk

Stir into saucepan and cook over medium heat until thickened.

15-1/2 oz. can salmon, drained with skin and bones removed

Stir into above mixture.

Cook, stirring occasionally.

Serve hot in soup bowls.

Leftovers can be frozen.

Creamy Broccoli Soup

Serves 6

1 Tbsp. safflower oil 3/4 cup onion, chopped	Sauté for 8 minutes.
1 cup water 6 vegetable or chicken bouillon cubes	Add bouillon to water to dissolve.
1 lb. broccoli, chopped 2 cups potatoes, diced 3/4 cup carrots, sliced 1 tsp. thyme 1 tsp. celery seed 1/4 tsp. marjoram 1/4 tsp. pepper	Bring to a boil. Simmer covered until vegetables are tender. Drain and add onions.
3 cups low fat milk 1/2 cup plain yogurt	Add to vegetables. Simmer 15 minutes. Serve hot in soup bowls.

Vegetable and Beef Stew

Serves 6

3 lbs. chuck, cut into bite size pieces 5 Tbsp. vegetable oil 1 cup green pepper, chopped 1 cup onion, chopped	Sauté until meat is brown. Set aside.
3/4 cup celery, chopped 12 oz. beef broth 1/2 cup water 8 oz. can tomatoes 1 clove garlic, finely chopped 1/4 tsp. pepper 1 bay leaf 1/8 tsp. thyme 6 small red potatoes, chopped 8 medium carrots, diced 1/2 cup pearl onions	Mix together. Place in large saucepan. Simmer 1 hour.
2 Tbsp. white flour 2 Tbsp. water	Mix together. Add to thicken stew. Simmer 35 minutes.

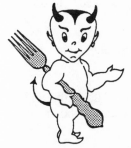

10. Salads and Salad Dressings

Introduction to Produce

Sometimes the thought of eating carrots or salads can seem boring. Eating the same food certainly can be boring, but there's nothing boring about produce. The produce department has one of the largest varieties of fresh fruit and vegetables. Alongside the carrots and lettuce there are some foods you've never been introduced to.

We have listed a few common and not so common vegetables. Try to keep an open mind and be adventurous and taste a few different varieties. Don't let their somewhat unusual appearance stop you from trying. It's the best way to find out if you like them.

When you are selecting produce here are a few tips that will help. Avoid produce that looks painted and waxed. If you can buy local produce it will be fresher than out-of-state produce that has to travel. Spraying with fungicides and waxes is more likely to be used to keep out-of-state produce fresh during travel. Frozen vegetables can also be a good buy. Vegetables that are stored in a clear package are a good way to see what you are buying.

Arugala is good if you like things with a pungent hot flavor with jagged dark green leaves. This vegetable can be used raw or added to soups or stir fry for a little zip or cooked and eaten like spinach.

Belgian endive looks like a cigar made from light colored yellow leaves. It has a stronger flavor than lettuce. It tastes good in soups or stir fried alone or with other vegetables. For added interest and flavor, mix with other salad greens.

Burdock root is a root vegetable that is long and slender. It seems to add a good texture and fiber to a dish. It's cooking time is about 12 minutes longer than most vegetables. Do not peel; just scrub the burdock.

Chayote is a squash and has a light green rind. It is similar to winter squash and is delicious baked, stir fried, or steamed.

Daikon is a white radish. It is good in salads that need a little zip. When used raw, it has a hot taste, but when cooked it develops a delicate sweet flavor.

Endive has rather course leaves that are curly and edges that are dark green with a light yellow stem. Endive is also called chicory and is good in salads or slightly cooked.

Escarole has large flat leaves and can be used in salads or slightly cooked. It adds a nice variety to a salad.

Jerusalem artichokes have a brown skin and don't look like an artichoke. They can be used like potatoes and even in salads.

Kohlrabi is related to the cabbage family and is similar to a turnip. The bulbs and green tops can be used in salads. The bulbs can be stir fried or steamed and have a mild flavor.

Parsnips are related to the carrot family and look like white carrots. They have a sweet and nutty flavor and taste good in soups and stews.

Rutabagas have a sweet tasting, rather nutty flavor. They are round and have a light yellow and brown skin. They taste great shredded on salads or used in casseroles or stews.

Shiitake mushrooms are used in Oriental and Western dishes. They are large chewy mushrooms and have a delicious flavor. Use in soups, stews, or stir fry.

Spaghetti squash is a yellow oblong shaped squash that can be baked or steamed. Its texture is long and stringy like spaghetti and it has a sweet flavor. Kokkaido squash is the sweetest of all squashes.

Taro root is a staple used in Japan and New Zealand. It looks like and can be used like a potato. The skin may be bitter, so remove after cooking.

Cauliflower Salad

Serves 8-10

1 head lettuce
1 head cauliflower
1 red onion, cut into rings
1/4 cup bacon bits

Dressing

1-1/2 cups light salad dressing
1/2 cup Parmesan cheese
1/4 cup sugar

Tear lettuce into pieces, break cauliflower into florets, layer all ingredients in a large salad bowl.

Mix together. Pour over the above ingredients. Cover the bowl and place in the refrigerator for a few hours or overnight. Stir before serving.

Green Bean Salad

Serves 8-10

3 lbs. green beans
1 medium red onion, sliced
1/4 cup olive oil
1/3 cup red wine vinegar
1/4 tsp. tarragon
1 tsp. salt
1 tsp. prepared mustard
1/2 tsp. pepper

Cook beans and onions tender crisp and drain.

Mix remaining ingredients together. Stir into beans and onions. Marinate in the refrigerator 2 hours.

This salad can be put in a tightly closed container and kept in the refrigerator for 5-6 days.

Cabbage Salad

Serves 10-12

7 cups cabbage, shredded or chopped
1 green pepper, diced
1/2 cup carrots, sliced or shredded

Layer in a large bowl.

1/2 cup white vinegar
1/2 cup vegetable oil
3/4 cup sugar
1/2 tsp. salt

Bring to a boil and pour over the vegetables.

Let stand in the refrigerator a few hours. Mix and serve.

Will keep a couple of weeks in the refrigerator.

The salad may be put in cartons and frozen.

Garlic and Herb Vegetable Salad

Serves 10-12

1 head cauliflower
1 bunch broccoli
1 lb. green beans
1 lb. carrots

Break cauliflower and broccoli into florets. Cut beans and slice carrots. Cook until tender crisp. Rinse with cold water. Drain and put in a large bowl.

1 cup vegetable oil
1 cup wine vinegar
1 clove garlic, minced
2 Tbsp. lemon juice
1/2 tsp. each paprika, dill, and pepper
1 Tbsp. Worcestershire sauce

Whisk together and pour over the vegetables. Cover and place in the refrigerator.

Wilted Lettuce Salad

Serves 4-6

3/4-1 lb. leaf lettuce	Wash and drain well. Tear into pieces. Place in salad bowl.
1/4 cup white vinegar **1/4 cup vegetable oil** **1/4 cup sugar** **1/4 tsp. salt** **Dash pepper**	Mix together in a saucepan. Bring to a boil. Pour over lettuce.
1/4 red onion	Cut into rings.
1/4 cup bacon bits	Toss with above ingredients. Serve at once.

Three Bean Salad

Serves 6-8

16 oz. can green beans **16 oz. can wax beans** **16 oz. can red kidney beans**	Drain and pour into a large bowl.
1/2 cup green pepper, chopped **1/2 cup onion, chopped**	Add to the above ingredients.
3/4 cup vinegar **1/4 cup vegetable oil** **1/2 scant cup sugar** **1 Tbsp. salt (optional)**	Mix together well. Pour over vegetables. Cover and let stand overnight in the refrigerator.

Oriental Spinach Salad

Serves 10-12

2 bags fresh spinach	Wash well and drain. Tear into pieces and put into a large salad bowl.
16 oz. can bean sprouts, drained 2 small cans water chestnuts, drained and sliced 1/4 cup bacon bits (soybean bits)	Mix together and add to spinach.
2 tsp. salt (optional) 1 cup vegetable oil 1/2 cup sugar 1/3 cup catsup 1/4 cup vinegar 1 Tbsp. Worcestershire sauce 1 medium onion, chopped	Mix in the blender. Stir into dressing. Pour over spinach when ready to serve.

Spinach Salad
with Lemon Dressing

Serves 10-12

2 - 10 oz. bags spinach 1 medium head lettuce 2 small Belgian endives (optional) 1/2 lb. medium mushrooms, sliced thin	Wash well and drain. Tear greens into pieces. Put in large bowl.
1 large lemon - 1/4 cup juice	Grate 2 tsp. peel.
2/3 cup vegetable oil 2 tsp. sugar 1 tsp. salt 1 tsp. dry mustard 1/4 tsp. course ground black pepper 1 tsp. fresh or dried chives, chopped	Whisk together. Add lemon peel. Keep in a covered jar in the refrigerator until ready to serve.

Needless to say, you don't have to make up a full batch of the greens unless you are serving 10-12 people.

Saucy Carrot Salad

Serves 8-10

2 lbs. carrots	Peel and slice in rounds. Cook until slightly tender. Drain and cool.
1/2 cup green pepper, chopped **1 small onion, peeled and sliced into rings**	Add to the carrots in a large bowl.
16 oz. can tomato soup **3/4 cup sugar** **1 cup vegetable oil** **3/4 cup vinegar** **1 tsp. salt** **1/4 tsp. pepper** **1 tsp. dry mustard**	Mix in a blender. Pour over the above ingredients. Cover and refrigerate until ready to serve. Keeps well in the refrigerator.

Carrot and Cauliflower Salad

Serves 6-8

1 medium head cauliflower	Break into bite size florets.
1/2 cup olive oil **1/2 cup red wine vinegar** **1/4 cup water** **2 medium cloves garlic, crushed** **1/4 tsp. salt** **1/4 tsp. pepper** **2 bay leaves**	Combine and add to cauliflower in a saucepan. Bring to boil and simmer 10 minutes.
1/2 cup onion, chopped **1/3 cup parsley, minced** **1/2 tsp. basil** **1 cup carrots, grated**	Add to cauliflower. Place in serving bowl and chill. Toss before serving.

Fresh Pineapple Salad

Serves 4-6

1-1/2 cups crushed pineapple
1 banana, sliced
1/2 cup strawberries, grapes, or apple
  chunks
1/3 cup raisins
1/4 cup orange juice, unsweetened
1/4 cup coconut, shredded

Mix together all ingredients.

Great on top of pancakes or as a dessert or snack over yogurt.

Cucumber Salad

Serves 4-6

1 cup red wine vinegar
4 tsp. honey

Mix in saucepan and heat until warm.

5 medium cucumbers, sliced
1 tsp. salt
1/4 tsp. pepper
1 tsp. dill weed
1/2 cup onion, chopped

Mix together and pour warm mixture
over cucumber mixture.
Refrigerate.

Beet Salad

Serves 6-8

10 beets

Boil whole and chop into bite size
pieces.

1/2 cup cider vinegar
1 medium clove garlic, crushed
3 tsp. honey

Mix together and add to beets.
Let stand 20 minutes.

1/2 cup onion, chopped
2 whole scallions, minced
2 medium cucumbers, chopped
1 hard boiled egg, chopped

Mix all ingredients and add to the beet
mixture.

Serve cold.

For more color you can add 1/3 cup corn.

Zucchini Salad

Serves 4-6

1 small bunch romaine lettuce, torn

1 Tbsp. olive oil   Mix together and toss with lettuce.
1 medium zucchini, thin sliced
1/2 cup radishes, sliced
2 Tbsp. green onions, sliced
2 tsp. blue cheese
1 Tbsp. tarragon
1 clove garlic, minced
Dash pepper

Carrot and Raisin Salad

Serves 4-5

3 cups carrots, grated   Combine.
1/2 cup raisins, chopped
1/4 cup almonds, slivered
2 Tbsp. parsley
1/4 cup celery, diced
1/4 cup onion, diced

Dressing

4 Tbsp. vegetable oil   Combine ingredients and whisk until
2 Tbsp. lemon juice   creamy.
1 tsp. rice syrup
                                         Toss with salad.

Mandarin Spinach Salad

Serves 4-6

4 cups spinach, torn into bite size
  pieces
1/2 cup cucumber, chopped
1/2 cup mandarin oranges, drained
8 ripe olives, chopped

Combine all ingredients and toss.

Sprinkle with sesame seeds if desired.

Creamy Cucumber Salad

Serves 4-6

4 large cucumbers, peeled

Cut into bite size pieces.

2 cups low fat yogurt
2 tsp. lemon juice
1/2 tsp. salt
Dash pepper
2 cloves garlic, minced
1 Tbsp. olive oil
2 Tbsp. parsley

Mix together and add to cucumbers.

Refrigerate before serving.

Onion and Tomato Savory Salad

Serves 4

4 small Spanish onions, sliced
1/4 cup water

Place on bottom of greased casserole
dish. Bake 15 minutes.

1 Tbsp. margarine or vegetable oil
1-1/2 cups mushrooms, sliced

Mix together and place on top of onions.

5 medium tomatoes, sliced

Layer on top of mushrooms.

1/3 cup dry bread crumbs

Sprinkle over salad.

Bake at 325°F for 30 minutes until
brown.

Mustard Dressing

2 Tbsp. Dijon mustard
1/4 cup white vinegar
1/2 cup olive oil
1/4 cup low fat milk
Dash salt
Dash cayenne
Dash black pepper

Combine and mix well.

Sweet and Sour Dressing

1/2 cup white vinegar
1/2 cup vegetable oil
3/4 cup sugar
1/2 tsp. salt

Mix together.
Heat to a boil.
Use hot or cold.

Celery Seed Dressing

2/3 cup sugar
1 tsp. dry mustard
1 tsp. paprika
1 tsp. celery seed
1/4 tsp. salt

Combine.

1/3 cup honey
1/3 cup vinegar
1 Tbsp. lemon juice
1 tsp. onion, chopped

Combine with above ingredients in blender.
Blend well.

1 cup vegetable oil

Add slowly to the above while blending.
Store in covered container in the refrigerator.

Sesame and Orange Dressing

1 cup orange juice
1/2 cup vegetable oil
1 Tbsp. tamari sauce
1 Tbsp. sesame seeds
1 clove garlic, crushed
1/2 tsp. dry mustard
1/2 tsp. dill weed

Combine and mix well.

French Dressing

1-1/2 cups vegetable oil
1 cup catsup
3/4 cup vinegar
2 Tbsp. lemon juice
1 small onion, cup up
1 tsp. celery salt
3/4 cup sugar
3 tsp. horseradish
1 tsp. paprika

Place all ingredients in a blender and blend well.

Makes one pint.

Pour into a jar with a screw top and keep in the refrigerator.

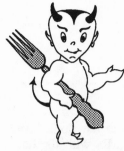

11. Hot and Cold Sauces

Sauces don't have to be loaded with fat to taste good. Most foods reach a **flavor point.** This is when the addition of more fat doesn't add to the flavor, just to the fat content. This is similar to boiling water: once you bring the water to its **boiling point** there's nothing more you can do.

It is by thickening your sauces with flour and cold water or low fat milk that you can create a low fat sauce that has a wonderful creamy texture and flavor. We call this FLOUR POWER.

You can use unbleached white flour, corn starch, arrowroot or kuzu for thickening sauces. When using arrowroot, kuzu or corn starch, use 1/2 the amount required for flour and slowly dissolve in cold water, and add to heated mixture while stirring. By adding a dash of saffron, garlic, basil, and thyme to your white sauce you can create a wonderful hollandaise sauce.

You will find our standard recipe in this section for making thick, medium, and thin sauces. In all our sauce recipes we have applied moderation while still keeping a fabulous flavor. We want to keep your taste buds happy! We have included hot and cold sauces that will give zest and a touch of elegance to meat, fish, vegetables, and even fruits.

Saffron Sauce

1 cup low fat milk

Heat.

2 Tbsp. flour
2 Tbsp. margarine
Dash of salt and pepper

Melt margarine. Stir in the flour. Add the salt and pepper. Mix with the hot milk. Cook and stir until thickened.

1/4 tsp. saffron
Pinch of basil and thyme (optional)

Stir into the above sauce. Serve over beef tenderloin or baked fish.

Seafood Sauce

1 cup low fat milk
1 clove garlic

Rub saucepan with garlic. Heat the milk.

2 Tbsp. flour
2 Tbsp. margarine
Dash of salt and pepper

Melt the margarine. Stir in the flour. Add salt and pepper. Mix with the milk. Cook and stir until thickened and smooth.

1/2 cup catsup
3 Tbsp. Worcestershire sauce

Add to the above ingredients.

Serve over lobster, shrimp, or baked fish.

Hollandaise Sauce

2 medium eggs or egg substitute
2 tsp. lemon juice
3 Tbsp. low fat milk

Whisk together and heat until slightly thickened.

2 tsp. Dijon mustard
Dash red pepper

Whisk into the above ingredients. Beat until thickened.

1 Tbsp. margarine

Whip into the above ingredients until smooth.

This sauce may be cooked on top of the stove or in the microwave.

To microwave, cooking on high, whisk after each 1/2 minute until desired thickness is obtained.

Nutmeg Sauce

2/3 cup honey
1 Tbsp. unbleached white flour

Mix together.

2/3 cup boiling water

Slowly add to honey mixture.
Whisk thoroughly.

1 Tbsp. margarine or vegetable oil
1 tsp. nutmeg
1 Tbsp. lemon juice

Add to above mixture.
Heat for 2 minutes.

Fruit Sauces

Serve over fruit, ice cream, yogurt, baked apples, waffles, or pancakes placed in dessert cups.

Raspberry Sauce

1-1/2 cups raspberries
1/3 cup honey
2 tsp. orange rind, grated
1/3 cup orange juice

Mix together.

Lemon Sauce

2 cups sesame tahini
1-1/2 cups buttermilk
1 medium clove garlic, crushed
1/2 cup fresh lemon juice
1/3 cup scallions, minced
1/3 cup parsley, minced
Dash salt
Dash paprika
1/2 tsp. cumin
1/4 tsp. tamari

Blend all ingredients together.

Great as salad dressing, added to sautéed vegetables, or served over fish.

Basic White Sauce

Thin

1 Tbsp. margarine, melted
1 Tbsp. flour

Mix together.

1 cup low fat milk, hot
Dash salt
Dash pepper

Add to the above.
Cook and stir until thickened.

If using the microwave, cook on high.
Stir every 30 seconds.
Cook until thickened.

Medium

2 Tbsp. margarine, melted
2 Tbsp. flour

Mix together.

1 cup low fat milk
Dash salt
Dash pepper

Add to the above.
Cook and stir until thickened.

Thick

3 Tbsp. margarine, melted
3 Tbsp. flour

Mix together.

1 cup low fat milk
Dash salt
Dash pepper

Add to the above.
Cook and stir until thickened.

Variations of Basic White Sauce

1 cup medium white sauce **3 Tbsp. catsup**	Mix together.

1 cup medium white sauce **1/2 cup grated low fat cheddar cheese**	Mix together.

1 cup medium white sauce **3-4 Tbsp. prepared horseradish** **1/8 tsp. saffron** **1 tsp. parsley**	Mix together.

Basic White Sauce
(very low fat)

1 cup low fat milk, cool **2 Tbsp. flour**	Whisk together. Cook and stir until thickened.

This sauce can be made with the same variations as the traditional white sauce.

Nacho Sauce

1-1/2 cups onion, chopped
2 large cloves garlic, crushed
2 Tbsp. olive oil

Sauté 5 minutes.

1/4 cup whole wheat flour

Add to above.
Sauté for 10 minutes.

1/3 cup coriander
1/3 cup cumin
1/3 cup cayenne
1 medium bell pepper, chopped
3 large tomatoes, chopped
1-1/2 cups low fat Monterey Jack
   cheese, grated
Dash pepper
2 cups water
2 tsp. sugar

Add all ingredients to sauté.
Cover and simmer 2 hours, stirring
frequently.

Serve hot so cheese will be melted.

Freeze some for later.

Use over chicken, chips, raw or cooked
vegetables, beans or rice.

Basic Tomato Spaghetti Sauce

1/4 cup onions, chopped
1 Tbsp. vegetable oil

Sauté in deep frying pan.

7 oz. tomato paste
1 can water
8 oz. can tomato sauce
1 can water
16 oz. can tomatoes, cut up
1 can water
2 cloves garlic, minced
1/4 tsp. salt
1/8 tsp. pepper
2 tsp. mixed Italian herbs or 1 tsp.
   oregano
1/2 tsp. basil
1/2 tsp. thyme

Add to the sauté.
Simmer until desired thickness.

Sauce with Tiny Shrimp

3/4 cup white sauce
1/4 to 1/2 cup tiny shrimp
1/4 tsp. saffron
1/4 tsp. parsley
Dash paprika
Dash salt
Dash pepper

Mix together.

Try this served over Fish Rolls with Corn Bread Stuffing on page 61.

Quick Cold Sauces

Horseradish

1/2 cup light mayonnaise
4 Tbsp. low fat milk
1-2 Tbsp. prepared horseradish
Dash paprika
Dash salt
Dash pepper

Whisk together.

Good served with beef or fish.

Dill

1/2 cup light mayonnaise
4 Tbsp. low fat milk
1 Tbsp. dried dill or 2 Tbsp. fresh dill,
   chopped
Dash salt
Dash pepper

Whisk together.

Good with fish.

Tartar Sauce

1/2 cup light mayonnaise
4 Tbsp. low fat milk
2-3 Tbsp. sweet pickle relish
Dash paprika
Dash salt
Dash pepper

Whisk together.

Good with fish.

Red Shrimp Sauce

1/2 cup catsup
1 Tbsp. onion, chopped
1 Tbsp. Worcestershire sauce
1/8 tsp. tabasco
Dash garlic powder
Dash salt
Dash pepper

Stir together.

Serve with shrimp or fish.

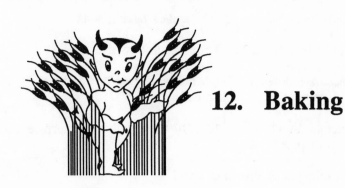

12. Baking

Cooking Trivia

Once the surface of bread is brown, it can't expand anymore.

Bread is done when it sounds hollow when tapped.

Bread, muffins, and biscuits are done when sides shrink away from the pan.

The browning of bread is due to the chemical change, which gives off the aroma.

For grains to be considered enriched they must contain thiamin, riboflavin, niacin, and iron.

White flour is just endosperm and is absent the bran and germ.

Grade A eggs are the best. B and C are less acceptable because of their thinner egg whites.

If indentation made by inserting two fingers into dough remains, the rising process is complete.

Unbleached flour should be aged naturally to avoid using a chemical bleaching agent.

There are 3 types of wheat -- hard, soft and durum wheat. All-purpose flour is a blend of hard and soft wheat.

Hard wheat is high in gluten, which is a protein that stretches to form an elastic texture and causes the product to rise.

If you mix or knead too much, you produce more gluten and you'll end up with a hard product.

Baking a product with bran prevents gluten from forming, and you'll get a product that is flat.

Rye flour is low in gluten and needs to be combined with wheat flour to improve rising ability.

Quick breads are leavened chemically with baking powder and/or baking soda.

Yeast breads are leavened biologically by yeast and take more time to rise.

In yeast breads, the major rising occurs before the dough bakes. Yeast breads are chewier and durable, not cakey and crumby like quick breads.

Rising still occurs when you refrigerate dough overnight. Oil the dough's top surface and place in a large bowl. Cover with plastic wrap.

Average kneading time is 15 to 20 minutes of vigorous work.

Bread rises quicker at a higher altitude and should be refrigerated to slow down this process. The warmer your kitchen, the faster dough will rise.

Store whole grain flour in your refrigerator. Keep cool and dry.

Too much salt and oil interferes with the yeast and formation of gluten strands.

Sugar is not only a sweetener but also a tenderizer because it decreases the strength of gluten stands.

Salt helps gluten stretch, and high gluten will give bread a high volume.

Non-wheat flours like soy flour, rice flour, corn flour, barley flour, and buckwheat flour have no gluten and should be combined with 3/4 cup wheat flour per 1/4 cup flour of your choice.

Buckwheat is not a grain but a member of the rhubarb family. Roasted buckwheat is known as kasha and has a nutty flavor.

Triticale is a hybrid developed by crossing wheat and rye; it is high in protein.

Bulgar is cracked wheat berries and is a great substitute for rice.

Self-rising flour is a combination of baking powder, salt, and flour.

Yeast requires sugar, warmth, and moisture to become activated and produce carbon dioxide needed to make the product rise.

Whole wheat pastry flour is a great substitute for regular pastry flour.

Durum wheat would not be used for cakes, pies, etc.   It is used to make pasta and is high in gluten (protein).

Semolina is durum flour with the bran and germ removed.

Soft wheats include pastry flour and cake flour. All provide a light product with less protein than hard wheat.

Eggs are an important leavening agent, as well as aiding in stirring and creaming fats and sugars into the food.

Higher quality flours help the dough to hold more water, thereby giving it strength and allowing it to stretch further.

Sourdough breads are made with a special sourdough culture responsible for their tangy, sour flavor.

Graham flour (coarser whole wheat ground) is named after Sylvester Graham, who was a believer in eating bran and gave his name to the graham cracker.

An unshortened cake like angel food will not rise if you grease the pan.

To cut down on cholesterol when baking -- use 1 Tablespoon vegetable oil for every egg and use some baking powder or soda as your leavening agent.

If you are using free flowing brown sugar, when measuring, don't pack it in -- sprinkle it in.

Rhubarb Muffins

12 muffins

4 oz. vegetable oil
1 cup sugar
1/4 tsp. vanilla
1 egg or egg substitute

Mix together.

2 cups white flour
4 tsp. baking powder
1/4 tsp. salt (optional)
1 cup low fat milk

Combine with above ingredients and stir well.

2 cups rhubarb, chopped

Mix into above ingredients.

Grease muffin tins or line with paper cups. Fill cups about 2/3 full. Bake at 400° for 30 minutes.

Bran Muffins

12 muffins

2 cups all bran
1-1/4 cups low fat milk

Mix and let stand until cereal is soft.

1 egg or egg substitute
1/4 cup vegetable oil

Add to above mixture and beat well.

1-1/4 cups flour
1 Tbsp. baking powder
1/2 tsp. salt (optional)
1/2 cup sugar

Add to above ingredients and stir only until combined.
Pour into muffin pans sprayed with non-stick cooking spray or lined with muffin papers.

Bake at 400°F for 20 minutes.

You may also add a few walnuts or raisins.

Bran Muffins with Honey

12 muffins

1 cup raw bran

1 cup unbleached white flour	Sift together.
1/4 tsp. salt	Add to bran.
1 tsp. baking soda	

1 cup low fat milk	Mix together.
1 medium egg or egg substitute	Add to dry ingredients.
1/3 cup orange blossom honey	
2 Tbsp. vegetable oil	

1/3 cup raisins Add to above mixture.

Pour muffin cups 2/3 full.
Bake at 350°F for 25 minutes.

Raisin Oat Muffins

12 muffins

1 cup unbleached white flour	Mix together.
3/4 cup whole wheat flour	
1/2 cup rolled oats	
1/4 tsp. salt	
1 tsp. baking soda	

3 Tbsp. margarine	Beat together.
2 Tbsp. honey	Add to dry ingredients.
1-1/2 cups low fat milk	
1 medium egg or egg substitute	

1/2 cup raisins Add to above.

Pour into muffin cups.
Bake at 375°F for 25 minutes.

Orange Yogurt Muffins

12 muffins

4 Tbsp. honey	Melt together.
4 Tbsp. margarine or vegetable oil	Remove from heat.
1 cup plain yogurt	Mix together.
1 medium egg or egg substitute	Add to honey mixture.
1/4 cup freshly squeezed orange juice	
1/2 tsp. orange rind, grated	
1 cup unbleached white flour	Mix together.
1 cup whole wheat flour	Add to above ingredients.
1/8 tsp. nutmeg	
1-1/2 tsp. baking soda	Pour into muffin cups.
1/4 tsp. salt	Bake at 375°F for 30 minutes.
1/3 cup walnuts, finely chopped	

Golden Corn Muffins

10-12 muffins

1 cup flour	Mix together.
1/2 cup yellow cornmeal	
1/2 cup sugar	
1 Tbsp. baking powder	
1/2 tsp. salt (optional)	
1 cup whole kernel corn, drained	Add to above ingredients.
	Toss to coat.
2 eggs or egg substitute	Beat with fork.
1/2 cup low fat milk	Beat into eggs.
1/2 cup vegetable oil	Add to corn mixture.
	Stir just until blended.
	Fill muffin cups sprayed with non-stick cooking spray or lined with paper liners 2/3 full.
	Bake at 400°F for 15-20 minutes.

Molasses Corn Muffins

12 muffins

1 cup yellow cornmeal

1 cup unbleached white flour	Sift together.
1/2 cup whole wheat flour	Add to cornmeal.
1/2 tsp. baking soda	
2 tsp. baking powder	
1/4 tsp. salt	

1-1/3 cups yogurt	Beat together.
1 medium egg or egg substitute	Add to dry ingredients.
2 Tbsp. margarine or vegetable oil	
1/8 tsp. cinnamon	Fill muffin cups 2/3 full.
4 Tbsp. molasses	Bake at 350°F for 25 minutes.

Spicy Carrot Muffins

12 muffins

2 cups unbleached flour	Mix together.
3 tsp. baking powder	
1 tsp. ground cinnamon	
1/2 tsp. salt	

1/2 cup honey	Blend together.
1 cup carrots, shredded	Mix with dry ingredients.
3/4 cup low fat milk	
1/3 cup vegetable oil	Fill muffin cups 3/4 full.
2 medium eggs or egg substitute	Bake at 400°F for 20 minutes.

Banana Bread

2 cups whole wheat flour 1 tsp. baking soda 1 tsp. baking powder 1 tsp. salt	Sift together dry ingredients in large bowl.
4 Tbsp. margarine or vegetable oil 1/2 cup honey	Cream together.
3 large bananas, mashed 2 eggs 1/2 cup low fat milk	Mix together. Add to margarine and honey, then to dry ingredients.
1/3 cup walnuts, chopped	Fold into above mixture.
	Pour into 9 x 5 inch greased loaf pan. Bake at 325°F for 55 minutes.

Cranberry Bread
(No Rising Required)

1-3/4 cups cranberries 1/3 cup margarine or vegetable oil 1/2 tsp. cinnamon 1/3 cup walnuts, minced	Mix together over medium heat in skillet for 8 minutes. Remove from heat.
1 cup whole wheat flour 1 cup unbleached white flour 2 tsp. baking powder 1/2 tsp. baking soda	Sift together. Add to hot mixture.
1/2 tsp. vanilla Dash nutmeg 1/4 cup honey 2 medium eggs or egg substitute 1/3 cup brown sugar	Beat together. Add to above ingredients. Spread into oiled or non-stick loaf pan. Bake at 350°F for 55 minutes.

Oatmeal Bread

(No Rising Required)

1 cup whole wheat flour 1 cup unbleached white flour 1-1/2 tsp. baking soda 1/2 tsp. baking powder 1/2 tsp. salt	Sift together.
1-3/4 cups rolled oats	Add to dry ingredients.
2 medium eggs or egg substitute 1/4 cup molasses 1-1/4 cups low fat milk 1/2 tsp. vanilla extract 3 Tbsp. margarine or vegetable oil 2 Tbsp. lemon juice 1 Tbsp. water	Mix together well. Add to dry mixture. Pour into loaf pan sprayed with non-stick cooking spray. Bake for 55 minutes at 350°F.

Soda Bread

3-1/2 cups flour 1/2 tsp. baking powder 3/4 cup sugar 1/2 tsp. salt	Mix together.
1/4 cup vegetable oil 1 egg or egg substitute	Whisk. Add to the above ingredients.
1 cup low fat buttermilk	Add to the above. Stir well.
1 cup raisins	Stir into batter. Knead lightly. Shape into a ball. Place on a baking tin sprayed with non-stick cooking spray. Bake at 350°F for 40-50 minutes.

Cinnamon Apple Bread

2 cups apples, grated
3-1/2 Tbsp. lemon juice

Mix together.

1/2 cup brown sugar
4 Tbsp. margarine or vegetable oil
1 medium egg or egg substitute

Mix together.
Add to apples.

1 cup unbleached flour
1 cup whole wheat flour
2 tsp. baking powder
1/2 tsp. baking soda
Dash salt
2 tsp. cinnamon

Sift together.

1/4 tsp. vanilla

Add to sifted ingredients.
Add to apple mixture.

Bake at 350°F for 45 minutes in an
oiled loaf pan or muffin cups.

Homemade Cheese Bread

2 cups unbleached white flour
2 tsp. baking powder
1/2 tsp. baking soda
1/8 tsp. salt

Sift together.

1-1/2 cups cottage cheese
2 medium eggs or egg substitute
5 Tbsp. low fat milk
1-1/2 Tbsp. honey
3 Tbsp. margarine or vegetable oil
1 Tbsp. dill seed, minced
1/2 Tbsp. rosemary

Mix together.
Slowly add to dry ingredients.

Spread into loaf pan.
Bake at 350°F for 40 minutes.

Molasses Oatmeal Bread

1 cup rolled oats 2 tsp. salt (optional) 2 Tbsp. vegetable oil 1/2 cup molasses	Stir together.
2-1/2 cups boiling water	Add to the above ingredients. Cool.
1 yeast cake or 1 pkg. dry yeast 1/2 cup warm water	Mix to dissolve yeast. Add to the above ingredients.
5-1/2 cups white flour (or use 1/2 wheat flour)	Add flour 1 cup at a time. Turn out onto a floured board. Knead in flour until smooth. (This dough tends to be a little sticky.) Put into a bowl sprayed with non-stick cooking spray. Cover with towel and let rise until double in size. Punch down. Divide in half. Place in 2 loaf tins sprayed with non-stick cooking spray. Cover with towel and let rise until double in size. Bake at 350°F for 30-40 minutes.

This bread makes an especially good toast and tuna salad tastes extra good on it.

Fresh Gingerbread

4 Tbsp. margarine or vegetable oil
3 Tbsp. ginger root, grated

Sauté 3 minutes.
Set aside.

1/2 cup honey
1/3 cup molasses
2/3 cup yogurt
1 medium egg or egg substitute

Beat together.
Add to sauté mixture.

1 cup whole wheat flour
1 cup unbleached white flour
1-1/2 tsp. baking soda
Dash salt
1/2 tsp. allspice
1/2 tsp. cinnamon
1/4 tsp. nutmeg

Sift together.
Add to above ingredients.

Bake at 350°F for 35 minutes in an
oiled 8 inch square pan.

Serve with vanilla yogurt or low fat
whipping cream.

Zucchini Spice Bread

2 cups zucchini, grated

1/3 cup honey
4 Tbsp. margarine or vegetable oil
2 medium eggs or egg substitute
1 tsp. vanilla

Mix together in blender.

1 cup unbleached white flour
1 cup whole wheat flour
1/2 tsp. salt
2-1/2 tsp. baking powder
1/4 tsp. ginger
1/4 tsp. nutmeg
1/2 tsp. allspice
1/2 tsp. cinnamon

Sift together.
Slowly add grated zucchini and honey
mixture.

Bake at 350°F for 40 minutes.
Spread into an oiled loaf pan.
Raisins and nuts are optional.

Corn Bread

3/4 cup yogurt
1 Tbsp. honey
2 Tbsp. margarine, melted
1 egg or egg substitute
1/2 cup carrots, shredded

Mix together.

3/4 cup cornmeal
1/2 cup whole grain corn flour
1/2 tsp. baking soda
1/2 tsp. salt

Combine with above ingredients.

Spray square baking pan with non-stick cooking spray. Pour batter into the pan. Bake at 375°F for 30 minutes.

Rosemary Whole Wheat Bread

2 loaves

Sponge

1 cup warm water
2 pkgs. active dry yeast
1/4 tsp. sugar
2 cups unbleached white flour

Prepare sponge and let dough rise completely as usual. Set aside.

3 cups whole wheat flour
1 tsp. salt
2 tsp. dried rosemary

Combine dry ingredients.

2 medium eggs or egg substitute
1/4 cup margarine
2 Tbsp. warm water

Beat together.
Add to dry ingredients.

Add to sponge.
Do usual kneading, rising, and punching, etc.
Bake risen loaf in oiled loaf pan at 375°F for 60 minutes.
Top with sesame seeds.

Can be frozen.

Butternut Squash Bread

Sponge

1 cup warm water
2 pkgs. active dry yeast
1/4 tsp. sugar
2 cups unbleached white flour

Prepare sponge and let dough rise completely as usual. Set aside.

2 cups butternut squash, baked until soft

Scoop out inside.
Let cool.

4 Tbsp. orange honey
1/4 cup margarine, melted
1 tsp. salt
2 tsp. cinnamon
1/2 tsp. cloves

Mix together.
Add to squash.

4 cups unbleached white flour
2 cups whole wheat flour

Mix together.
Add to above ingredients.

Add all ingredients to sponge.
Do usual kneading, rising, punching, etc.
Place dough in oiled loaf pan.
Bake risen loaves at 375°F for 60 minutes.

Can be frozen.

Use leftover squash for a side dish at next dinner.

Sunflower Seed Bread

Sponge

1 cup warm water 2 pkgs. active dry yeast 1/4 tsp. sugar 2 cups unbleached white flour	Prepare sponge and let dough rise completely as usual. Set aside.
1/4 cup margarine 4 Tbsp. honey 2 tsp. salt 3/4 cup sunflower seeds	Combine in skillet. Heat for 10 minutes. Let cool.
1-1/4 cups unbleached white flour 2 cups whole wheat flour	Mix together. Add to above ingredients.
1 cup low fat milk	Add to above ingredients.
	Add all ingredients to sponge. Do usual kneading, rising, punching, etc. Place risen loaves in oiled loaf pan. Bake at 375°F for 60 minutes. Freeze one for later.

Dill Bread

3/4 cup warm water
1 tsp. sugar
1 pkg. dry yeast

Mix together to dissolve yeast.
Let stand 10 minutes.

2 cups low fat cottage cheese

Cream in blender or food processor.

1 Tbsp. vegetable oil
1/4 cup onion, chopped

Sauté onions in oil.

2 tsp. salt (optional)
2 eggs or egg substitute

Beat lightly.
Add to the above ingredients.

2 Tbsp. dried dill
5 cups flour

Add dill and 1/2 of flour to the above.
Mix well.
Add remaining flour.
Mix well.

Put on floured board.
Knead.
Place in a bowl sprayed with non-stick
cooking spray.
Cover with a towel and let rise until
double in size.

Punch down.
Divide in half.

Put in two 9 x 5 loaf pans sprayed with
non-stick cooking spray.
Cover with a towel and let rise again
until double in size.

Bake at 350°F for 45-50 minutes.

Garlic Bread

1 loaf French bread	Slice diagonally.
1/2 cup margarine, softened or vegetable oil	Combine ingredients and stir well. Spread mixture on bread.
1 clove garlic, crushed	
3 Tbsp. Parmesan cheese, grated	Place bread slices on ungreased baking sheet.
1/4 tsp. pepper	
Dash red pepper	Bake at 350°F for 10 minutes.

Baking Powder Biscuits

2 cups flour	Mix together.
4 tsp. baking powder	
1 tsp. salt (optional)	
4 Tbsp. vegetable oil	Whip together.
3/4 cup low fat milk	Stir into dry ingredients.
	Form biscuits in size desired with hands and place on a baking sheet sprayed with non-stick cooking spray or knead dough for 20 seconds, pat or roll 1/2 inch thick, cut into rounds.
	Bake at 450°F for 10-15 minutes.
	(Hand formed biscuits are lighter.)

Whole Wheat Buttermilk Biscuits

1 cup unbleached white flour
1 cup whole wheat flour
2 tsp. baking powder
1/2 tsp. baking soda
1/2 tsp. salt

Sift together dry ingredients.

1 medium egg or egg substitute
2/3 cup low fat buttermilk
1/3 cup margarine, melted

Beat together.
Combine with dry ingredients.

Knead dough briefly until smooth.
Roll to 1/4 inch thickness.
Cut using favorite cookie cutters.
Bake at 450°F for 10-12 minutes.

Biscuits for Shortcake

2 cups flour
4 tsp. baking powder
1 tsp. salt (optional)
2 Tbsp. sugar

Mix together.

4 Tbsp. vegetable oil
3/4 cup low fat milk

Whisk together.
Add to dry ingredients.

Form biscuits in size desired with hands
and place on a baking sheet sprayed with
non-stick cooking spray or knead dough
for 20 seconds, pat or roll 1/2 inch thick,
cut into rounds.
Bake at 450°F for 12-15 minutes.

Basic Noodles

2 cups flour
1/2 tsp. salt
2 eggs or egg substitute, well beaten
2 Tbsp. warm water

Place flour and salt on a pastry board or in a large bowl.
Make a well in the center.
Add the egg and water.
Work flour into the egg mixture.
Add more water if necessary to make the dough workable.
Knead until smooth.

Divide dough in half.
Let rest 30 minutes covered.

Roll out as thin as possible.
Cut into any desired shape.

It is best to let them dry well before using.

To cook, drop them in boiling water.
Cook 12-15 minutes.

Popover Yorkshire Pudding

Serves 4-6

1/4 cup vegetable oil

Pour in 9 x 12 inch baking pan or individual popover cups.
Heat at 450°F for 10 minutes.

2 eggs or egg substitute

Beat until frothy.

7/8 cup low fat milk
1 Tbsp. margarine, melted

Add to eggs.

1 cup flour
1/4 tsp. salt

Stir slowly into liquid mixture.
Whisk until well blended - no longer.

Pour into hot pan or hot popover cups.
Bake at 450°F for 20 minutes.
Reduce heat to 350°F and bake an additional 15-20 minutes.

Cut loaf into squares and serve with roast beef and gravy.

Whole Wheat Waffles

1 cup whole wheat flour
1/4 cup unprocessed oat bran
2 tsp. baking powder
1/2 tsp. baking soda
1/4 tsp. ground nutmeg
1/8 tsp. ground cinnamon

Combine and stir well.

1 cup low fat buttermilk
1/4 cup unsweetened orange juice
2 Tbsp. vegetable oil
1 egg or egg substitute

Whisk. Add to the above ingredients.
Stir just until moistened.

Bake in waffle iron sprayed with non-stick cooking spray, or cook like pancakes.

Top with fresh fruit to serve.

Homemade Croutons

6 bread slices	Cut into 1/2 inch cubes
2 Tbsp. sesame seed oil Dash pepper 1/4 tsp. parsley 1/4 tsp. savory 1/4 tsp. oregano	Mix together. Sauté with bread cubes for 5 minutes. Place sautéed cubes on baking sheet. Bake at 300°F for 10 minutes.

Spinach Crust

2/3 lb. spinach, chopped very fine 2 Tbsp. margarine	Melt margarine in skillet. Add spinach. Heat until soft. Remove from heat.
2/3 cup unbleached white flour 1/2 cup wheat germ 1/4 tsp. salt 1/8 tsp. nutmeg	Mix together. Stir into spinach. Using a fork, mold crust into a 9 inch pie pan. Pat firmly with fingers. Pre-bake at 350°F for 15 minutes. Add meat or vegetables, if desired, as fillings.

Small Batch of Vegetable Oil Pie Crust

1-3/4 cups flour 1 tsp. salt (optional) 1/2 cup oil 3 Tbsp. cold water	Mix well. Roll between wax paper.

Pie Crust
(large amount)

5-1/2 cups flour **1 lb. shortening** **1 tsp. salt (optional)**	Blend together.
1 egg or egg substitute	Beat well in a cup.
2 tsp. vinegar	Add to egg.
Cold water	Add to above to make 1 cup. Mix well with dry ingredients.

This crust may be formed in amounts large enough for one crust, wrapped in wax paper, placed in a plastic bag and put in the freezer.

Thaw at room temperature or in the microwave on low setting 30 seconds to 1 minute.

It's great to have pie crust on hand.

Pie Crust
(large amount with unsaturated oil)

5 cups flour **1 tsp. salt (optional)**	Blend
1 egg or egg substitute **1 tsp. vinegar** **1/2 cup cold water** **1 cup vegetable oil**	Whisk. Add to flour. Mix well.

Roll out between wax paper.
This also may be separated in amounts large enough for one crust, wrapped in wax paper, placed in a plastic bag and frozen.

Crust made with oil is not as elastic as regular crust, so the amount needed for one crust is a little more.

Nut Crust

1/2 cup almonds, finely minced **4 Tbsp. margarine** **1-1/4 cups unbleached flour** **1/8 tsp. salt**	Combine in large bowl. Use pastry cutter to blend until firm.
5 Tbsp. cold water	Gradually add to dry mixture with fork. Roll out dough and form into 9 inch crust. Dough can be frozen for later use. Pre-bake at 350°F for 15 minutes. Add meat, vegetables, or fruit for filling to this versatile crust.

Crumb Crust

1 cup plain bread crumbs **1/4 cup whole wheat flour** **1/4 cup wheat germ** **3/4 cup rolled oats** **1/4 tsp. salt** **1/8 tsp. basil** **1/8 tsp. marjoram**	Mix together.
1/4 cup margarine, melted **2 Tbsp. warm water**	Drizzle into dry mixture and blend well with fork until mixture is uniform. Press mixture into 9 inch pie pan. Pre-bake at 350°F for 15 minutes. Fill with meat or vegetables if desired.

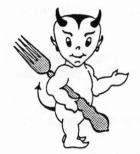

13. Kids' Recipes

Tips for Parents and Kids that Make Eating Fun!

You might be thinking it's time for a NEW APPROACH! Eating time can present a real challenge to parents. If children can learn to enjoy certain foods early, they will have a greater chance of becoming healthier eaters for life. Here are some tips that will help encourage eating and cooperation at mealtime.

Meals should be served on a regular schedule.

Make sure your child is in a comfortable chair, or eating can be too frustrating.

Don't coax them to eat. Serve small helpings and then remove their plate in 30 minutes. Don't battle it out.

Don't refer to your child as a fussy eater...they'll just live up to the label.

Refusal to eat can be the first sign indicating their need for independence. This is usually a brief power struggle. Simply ask your child to try everything; don't force him or her to finish everything.

Let kids help, by placing napkins on the table, or giving fun names to food. Try having each family member decide on a particular dish. When they see others respecting their food selection, they may be more willing to try the favorite of others in the family.

Don't use cakes and cookies as a reward. A dessert is part of a meal. Similar to reading their favorite book -- they start at the beginning, not the end.

Children have a very sensitive sense of taste. Stick to mild flavored foods.

Sometimes finger foods are a good idea. Silverware can be frustrating for children to use all the time.

Make sure your children are getting enough physical activity, to maintain a healthy appetite.

Children prefer foods served alone, rather than in casseroles, until they get older.

If your child's milk glass or pitcher is too large, it will discourage him or her from drinking.

Parents set an example. Whether or not parents want this role, it nevertheless is theirs. Children observe and usually will imitate those around them. Therefore, parents need to "Do as I say -- *and* as I do."

The kids' recipes in this chapter are designed to encourage participation, and are easy to prepare and inexpensive. Enjoy!

Peach Frosty

2 ripe peaches or 3 canned peach halves 2 cups low fat milk 1 banana 8 oz. plain yogurt 1/2 tsp. vanilla 5 ice cubes	Combine all ingredients in blender. Blend until smooth.

Pocket Surprise

2 slices turkey or chicken 1/4 cup mozzarella cheese, shredded 1 pickle, chopped 2 Tbsp. light mayonnaise	Mix together.
2 small pita bread pockets	Spoon mixture into pita pockets.

Kids love to put things in pockets, so let them be creative and add more to these pocket surprises.

Mini English Muffin Pizzas

4 English muffin halves, toasted

2 Tbsp. tomato sauce 1/4 cup mozzarella cheese, shredded 1/8 tsp. oregano Onion, chopped Parmesan cheese	Layer on top of muffins. Place in microwave 1-1/2 minutes or until cheese is melted.

Let your child add his or her favorite toppings.

Nutty Popcorn Balls

1/4 cup honey
1/4 cup water

Stir together over medium heat.

1/4 cup margarine
1 Tbsp. vanilla

Add to above ingredients.

1 quart popped popcorn
1 cup raisins
1 cup peanuts, chopped

Mix and add to other ingredients.

Roll into balls.

Cinnamon Honey Spread

2/3 cup apple butter
3-1/2 Tbsp. honey
1/2 tsp. ground cinnamon

Blend all ingredients.

Serve on bagels, waffles, pancakes, or toast.

Orange marmalade (unsweetened) could be used in place of apple butter.

Five Minute Soup

4 cups chicken broth
1/2 cup corn
1/2 cup carrots, cooked
1/2 cup lean turkey, shredded leftover

Heat all ingredients in broth.
Bring to a boil.

Serve with bagel, muffin, or whole wheat crackers.

Kid's like small oyster crackers to float in soup.

Alphabet Surprise

1 cup alphabet noodles 4 cups water	Boil until tender. Drain.
2 Tbsp. olive oil 1/2 cup tuna	Toss noodles in oil and tuna.
Cheese, Parmesan, Swiss or cheddar, shredded	Sprinkle over above.

Hawaiian Popcorn Delight

7 cups white popped popcorn 1/2 cup dried pineapple, chopped 1/4 cup nuts, chopped 1/4 dried papaya, chopped	Toss together all ingredients.
1/3 cup warm water 1/3 cup orange honey 1 tsp. salt 1-1/2 Tbsp. margarine or vegetable oil	Mix together and heat until melted. Pour over popcorn mixture. Press firmly in oiled pan. Refrigerate. Cut into squares.

Kids love them in their lunch box.

Banana Oatmeal Delight

1-1/2 cups water 1 Tbsp. orange juice 1/4 cup raisins	Bring to boil.
1 cup oatmeal	Add to boiling mixture. Turn off heat and stir constantly.
1/8 tsp. salt 1/2 banana, sliced 1 apple, pealed and diced	Add to oatmeal.

Crisp Rice Treats

1/2 cup honey 2 Tbsp. peanut butter 1 tsp. vanilla 1 tsp. sesame oil	Mix together. Warm over low heat.
3 cups crispy cereal	Add to warm mixture. Spread mixture in oiled 8 inch square pan. Let cool. Cut into squares.

Nuts, raisins or carob chips can be added.

Carob Banana Popsicles

4 bananas

Peel and cut in half.
Place on 8 popsicle sticks.

2 Tbsp. honey
3 Tbsp. warm water
1/3 cup carob chips

Mix together.
Melt over low heat.

Dip banana halves into syrup. Roll in nuts.

Freeze bananas.
Once frozen, wrap completely and place in freezer until ready to eat.

Apple-Cheese Pancakes

1 cup low fat cottage cheese
1-1/2 cups apples, grated
1/2 cup unbleached white flour
1/4 cup whole wheat flour
1 Tbsp. honey
1 Tbsp. sunflower seeds
1 tsp. cinnamon
Dash allspice
Dash nutmeg
Dash salt

Mix together.

4 eggs or egg substitute

Beat until firm.
Add to dry mixture.

Fry pancakes with non-stick cooking spray, safflower oil, or in a non-stick fry pan.

Serve with yogurt or fresh fruit.

Chocolate Syrup

1 oz. unsweetened chocolate
1/4 cup honey
1/8 tsp. salt
2 Tbsp. water

Heat in double boiler over low heat until chocolate is melted.
Remove from heat.

1-1/2 Tbsp. margarine
1/4 tsp. vanilla

Blend into chocolate mixture.

Yield 1/2 cup.
Serve over yogurt or banana slices.

Fresh Peanut Butter and Pear Spread

2 cups peanuts

Grind in blender about 1 minute.

1/4 cup vegetable oil

Add to ground peanuts 1 Tablespoon at a time while continuing to blend.

4 oz. canned pears, drained

Slowly add pears to blender 1 at a time.

Kids will love to spread this on bagels or graham crackers.

Zucchini Sandwich

1 medium zucchini, sliced
1/3 cup low fat cheddar cheese, grated
1 Tbsp. onion, chopped
4 slices 100% whole wheat bread, toasted

Microwave sandwich until cheese is melted.

Add fresh tomato slice to each sandwich.

Kids' Pizza

Easy Dough

1 pkg. dry yeast
1 tsp. sugar
1 cup warm water
1 Tbsp. vegetable oil
1 tsp. salt
3 cups unbleached white flour

Mix ingredients.
Knead dough.
Cover and let rise in warm place for 20 minutes.
Roll out dough and fit to pizza pan.
Bake dough at 350°F for 5 minutes.

Pizza Toppings

1/2 cup tomato sauce
2 small each yellow, red and green bell peppers
1/2 lb. ground turkey, rolled into small sausage balls
1 cup mozzarella cheese, shredded

Layer on dough.

Bake at 375°F for 15 minutes, until cheese melts and has golden brown crust.

Zucchini Scramble

Serves 4-5

1-1/4 cups zucchini, sliced
2 Tbsp. margarine or vegetable oil
2 Tbsp. onion, chopped
1/2 cup carrots, sliced

Sauté.

Dash pepper
Dash salt
1 Tbsp. flour
1/2 cup low fat milk

Heat milk.
Blend together in saucepan until sauce thickens.
Add to sauté.

1/4 cup cheddar cheese, grated
1/8 tsp. thyme

Add to thickened sauce.

2 tomatoes, cut into wedges

Add to sauce.

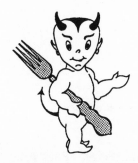

14. Snacks

People love to snack. However, somewhere along the way manufacturers confused snacks with desserts. Snacks should be nutritious and delicious. If you're tired of eating the same old thing, a snack can add some variety to your eating style and give you a nutritional boost. Snacking can help keep blood sugar stable, and can keep you feeling alert all day.

We recommend controlled snacking, not random snacking, which would be grabbing a giant sized bag of potato chips everyday at the Stop and Go. Potato chips are OK -- in moderation!

Many of the snacks we created can be eaten at home or away. Taking a snack to work is a great idea, especially if a microwave and small refrigerator are available. A couple of quick and simple snack ideas would be -- cinnamon toast with tea, or coffee, carrots and zucchini dipped in seasoned yogurt. Whole wheat crackers with tuna, pudding made with low fat milk, fresh fruit, and popcorn with a splash of honey.

Try some of our snack recipes at parties instead of the old standby chips and pretzels.

Cocobars

1 can crushed pineapple
1 medium egg or egg substitute

Beat egg. Stir in pineapple.

2 cups coconut
3/4 cup flour
1/4 cup wheat germ

Mix with above ingredients. Pour batter into an 8 inch pan sprayed with non-stick cooking spray.

Bake at 350°F for 40 minutes.

Cut into bars and serve.

Carrot and Raisin Salad

4 cups carrots, grated
1/2 cup raisins

Mix.

2 cups plain yogurt
1/4 tsp. vanilla

Whip together. Add to the raisin mixture. Stir and serve.

Cinnamon Meringue Cookies

3 large egg whites
1/4 tsp. cream of tartar

Whip egg whites until firm.
Add cream of tartar.

2 cups mixed chopped nuts
3 Tbsp. sugar
1/4 tsp. cinnamon

Fold into meringue.

Place in heaping tablespoons onto ungreased baking sheet.
Bake at 375° for 10 minutes or until golden brown.

Sweet Pea Guacamole

10 oz. frozen peas	Cook and drain.
1 jalapeño pepper	Place in the blender with the peas. Blend well.
1/4 cup olive oil **1-1/2 Tbsp. lemon juice** **1/4 tsp. cumin** **1/4 tsp. salt**	Add to the above ingredients. Blend well.
2 inch piece of red onion	Add onion and blend just enough to chop.
	Pour into a bowl. Serve as a dip with chips or crackers.

Graham Crackers

3/4 cup whole wheat flour **1/2 tsp. salt** **1/2 tsp. baking powder** **1/4 tsp. cinnamon**	Sift together and mix in bowl.
6 Tbsp. margarine **1/2 cup honey**	Blend and pour into dry ingredients. Place on well floured surface and roll dough to 1/8-inch thickness. Cut into rectangles 1-1/3 inch x 3 inches, then prick with a fork. Bake at 375°F on greased pan for 10 minutes.

Cottage Cheese Puffs

1 dozen

1 cup unbleached white flour
1/4 tsp. salt
1/4 tsp. marjoram
1/4 tsp. paprika

Mix dry ingredients together.

2/3 cup low fat cottage cheese
2 medium eggs or egg substitute
2 Tbsp. margarine or vegetable oil
1/4 cup water

Whip ingredients together.

Add flour mixture and stir well.

Place by tablespoonfuls onto baking sheet.

Bake at 375°F for 40 minutes or until brown.

Cheese Twists

2 cups whole wheat flour
1/4 tsp. paprika

Mix together.

1/3 cup margarine or vegetable oil
1 cup low fat cheddar cheese
1/2 cup cold water

Mix together.
Add to dry ingredients.
Blend until smooth.

Roll dough onto floured surface to 1/4 inch thickness.
Cut thin slices and twist.

Parmesan cheese, grated

Sprinkle twists with cheese.

Twists can be frozen and kept on hand for a snack.

Zucchini Cheese Nachos

2 medium zucchini

Slice and arrange on 9 inch pie pan.

1/4 tsp. onion powder
1/4 tsp. basil, crushed
1/4 tsp. oregano, crushed
3/4 cup low fat mozzarella cheese,
   shredded
1/3 cup pepperoni, chopped
4 tsp. Parmesan cheese, grated

Sprinkle on top of zucchini slices evenly.

Bake at 350°F for 10 minutes, until
cheese is melted.

Oatmeal Raisin Bars

2-1/3 cups whole wheat flour
2-1/2 cups rolled oats

Mix together.

1/2 cup safflower oil
1/3 cup honey
1 tsp. vanilla
1/8 tsp. salt

Mix together and add to dry ingredients.

1 cup raisins
1/3 cup hot water

Purée in blender.

Take 2/3 of oat mixture and press in
bottom of oiled 8 x 12 inch baking dish.

Spread puréed raisins on mixture.
Sprinkle remaining oat mixture on top.
Sprinkle chopped nuts on top if desired.

Bake at 350°F for 40 minutes.

Great for breakfast too!

Strawberry Oatmeal Bars

1/2 cup honey 1/3 cup margarine 1 tsp. vanilla extract	Blend together.
1 cup quick cooking oats, uncooked 3/4 cup unbleached white flour 1/4 cup 100% whole wheat flour 1/2 tsp. baking soda Dash salt	Combine. Add to margarine mixture. Press 2 cups of mixture into bottom of 8 inch square baking dish. Bake crust at 375°F for 8 minutes. Let cool.
10 oz. unsweetened fresh or frozen strawberries 1 Tbsp. honey 2 Tbsp. cornstarch 1/4 tsp. almond extract	Combine and spread over crust. Place remaining crust over strawberries. Bake at 375°F until top crust is golden brown.

Carob Brownies

1/4 cup unbleached flour	Set aside.
1/2 cup peanut butter 1 cup carob powder 1 cup vegetable oil 2/3 cup honey	Blend and add flour.
3 medium eggs or egg substitute 2 tsp. vanilla extract 1/2 cup mixed nuts, chopped	Mix together and add to flour mixture. Spread mixture in 9 inch square pan. Bake at 325°F for 35 minutes.

Chili Crab Dip

12 oz. carton low fat cottage cheese, drained 4 oz. light cream cheese	Blend in blender until creamy. Place in serving bowl. Chill.
1 cup chili sauce	Pour over cheese mixture when ready to serve.
6 oz. can crab meat, drained	Pour over the above.
	Serve with crackers.

Cucumber Dill Dip

1-1/2 cups low fat cottage cheese 2 medium cucumbers, peeled and chopped 1 Tbsp. lemon juice 2 Tbsp. green onion, chopped 1/2 tsp. dill weed 1/2 tsp. garlic	Mix together and chill. Great vegetable dip or sandwich spread in place of butter or margarine.

Ginger Dip

1/2 cup low fat plain yogurt 4 tsp. lime juice 1 Tbsp. honey 1/2 tsp. ground ginger 1/4 tsp. vanilla	Mix together and chill.
Dash nutmeg	Sprinkle over fruit.

Chutney Cheese Spread

**12 oz. carton low fat cottage cheese,
  drained
4 oz. light cream cheese**

Blend together in blender.

**1/4 cup mango chutney
1 tsp. curry
1/4 tsp. prepared mustard**

Stir into the cheese mixture.
Place in serving bowl.
Chill until ready to serve.

Serve with crackers or fresh vegetables.

Homemade Granola

**1 cup rolled oats, uncooked
1/4 cup nuts, chopped
1/3 cup wheat germ
1/3 cup sesame seeds
1/3 cup sunflower seeds
1/3 cup coconut, shredded**

Place ingredients in a large skillet.
Cook over medium heat, stirring
constantly, for 12 minutes. (Nuts should
begin to roast.)

**1/3 cup brown sugar
1/4 tsp. salt**

Add to nut mixture.
Continue to stir for 2-3 minutes.

Makes 3 cups.

Store in airtight container to keep its crunchy fresh taste.
Add to ice cream, yogurt, oatmeal, or any cereal, or use as a topping on or in muffins.

Cheerio Snack Mix

**4 cups Cheerios
1 cup dried apples, cut up
1/2 cup raisins
1/4 tsp. cinnamon**

Mix together in a snack bowl.

Makes a great afternoon snack!

Hawaiian Pineapple Pops

12 - 3 oz. paper cups
12 wooden sticks

1 can frozen orange juice concentrate	Blend together.
1 can low fat evaporated milk	Fill paper cups and freeze.
16 oz. low fat yogurt	
8 oz. can crushed pineapple	
1 Tbsp. honey	

Quick Fruit Cobbler

1 cup apples, chopped	Place in baking dish.
1/2 cup pears, chopped	
3 Tbsp. margarine, softened	Mix together until mixture is crumbly.
1/2 cup unbleached white flour	Spread over fruit.
1/2 cup rolled oats	
3 Tbsp. honey	
1/4 tsp. cinnamon	
2 Tbsp. raisins	Sprinkle over above mixture.
	Bake at 350°F for 25 minutes.
	Cool before serving.

Peanut Butter and Raisin Bars

2-1/2 cups granola	Mix together.
1/2 cup raisins	Add more peanut butter if needed.
1/2 cup water	
1/2 cup peanut butter	Roll into 1 inch round balls.
	Refrigerate until ready to eat.

Rice and Raisin Pudding

1-1/2 cups low fat milk	Heat until hot.
2 medium eggs or egg substitute **3 Tbsp. honey** **1/2 tsp. nutmeg** **1/4 tsp. cinnamon**	Combine and add to hot milk.
1/2 cup uncooked brown rice **1/2 cup raisins**	Add to above ingredients. Stir well. Cover and let simmer over medium heat for 30 minutes, stirring occasionally. Serve hot or cold topped with a cherry.

Great snack and kids love it!

Avocado and Pine Nut Salad

1 small head lettuce **1 medium tomato, chopped** **1 medium avocado, chopped** **1/3 cup pine nuts, toasted** **1/3 cup alfalfa sprouts** **1/3 cup onions, chopped**	Mix together. Use your favorite salad dressing or sprinkle with a little Parmesan cheese and lemon with pepper.

Garlic Toast

6 slices French bread

1 medium clove garlic, mashed **2 Tbsp. olive oil** **Dash pepper** **Dash rosemary**	Mix together and brush on both sides of bread slices. Bake at 450°F until toasty brown.

Apricot Walnut Bread

1 cup whole wheat flour
1 cup unbleached white flour

Mix together.

1 cup honey
1 tsp. baking soda
1/4 tsp. salt
1 egg or egg substitute
2 Tbsp. margarine or vegetable oil
1 tsp. vanilla
1 tsp. almond extract
1/2 cup walnuts, chopped
1 cup dried apricots (without sulfites),
  chopped

Mix together well.
Slowly add dry ingredients.

Bake at 375°F for 45 minutes.
Place mixture in 9 x 5 loaf pan sprayed
with non-stick cooking spray.

Ginger Pudding

4 cups low fat milk

Heat milk. Do not boil.

1/2 cup yellow cornmeal

Whisk together with milk.
Cook over medium heat, stirring
occasionally for 25 minutes until
thickened and smooth.

3/4 cup bran rice syrup
1/2 tsp. ground ginger
1 tsp. cinnamon
1/4 tsp. allspice
2 medium eggs or egg substitute

Mix together.
Add to cornmeal mixture.
Mix thoroughly.

Pour pudding into baking dish that has
been sprayed with non-stick cooking
spray.
Bake at 300°F for 1-1/2 hours.

Pumpkin Squares

2 medium eggs or egg substitute	Beat well.
1/2 cup honey 3/4 cup pumpkin, cooked and mashed 1 tsp. vanilla extract	Beat into egg mixture.
3/4 cup unbleached white flour 1 tsp. baking powder 1 tsp. ground cinnamon 1/2 tsp. ground ginger 1/4 tsp. salt 1/4 tsp. ground nutmeg	Combine in large mixing bowl. Add in egg and honey mixture. Stir well. Place batter in 9 inch square baking pan. Cut into squares. Let cool. Sprinkle with powdered sugar. Top with yogurt if desired.

Kashi and Honey

2 cups liquid 1 cup Kashi (seven grains and sesame)	Cook over medium heat for 25 minutes.
2 Tbsp. lavender honey 1 tsp. cinnamon 1 Tbsp. margarine	Add to cooked Kashi.

Apples and raisins can also be added if desired.

Butternut Squash with
Raisins and Cranberries

1 medium butternut squash	Cut in half and scoop out seeds. Bake at 375°F until tender. Scoop out and place in bowl.
3 medium apples, chopped **1/3 cup honey** **1-1/2 cups cranberries** **1/2 cup margarine** **Dash cinnamon** **Dash nutmeg**	Mix together. Add to squash. Place mixture in baking dish and heat. Sprinkle with chopped nuts.

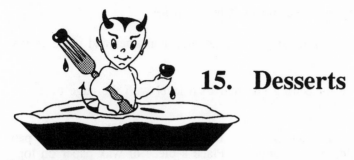

15. Desserts

Cooking Trivia

Before cutting: to extract more juice from lemons, limes, oranges, or grapefruits, place in microwave a few seconds, or roll on the counter top with the palm of your hand using some pressure to soften the pulp.

Use egg white only (no yolks) for unshortened cakes like chiffon, sponge, or angel food cakes.

To aid in chopping dried fruit, sprinkle with flour.

Chopping raisins will give more flavor to your product.

Cornstarch and arrowroot have twice the thickening power of flour.

When making whipped cream from low fat milk, use 1/4 of a teaspoon of cornstarch or cream of tartar to keep the cream firm.

The color of the eggshell is no indication of nutritional value. White eggs come from the white leghorn chicken, and the brown eggs are laid by larger breeds of hens called Rhode Island Reds. The brown eggs cost more because the Rhode Island Reds eat more and need more cage room.

When fresh fruits are cooked, they lose their semipermeable character and sugar enters the fruit.

Cooking in moist heat softens fibers, and adding sugar straightens fibers.

Do not roll pie crust again and again or it will not be flaky.

Too little water will make a crumbly crust.

There are different organic acids found in fruits: Malic acid is found in apples, tartaric acid in grapes, and citric acid in oranges.

Fats and sugars are tenderizers which shorten gluten strands, and if you reduce these too much your product will be as hard as a rock.

Pierce the bottom of your pie crust with a fork when it is to be filled after baking.

The more sugar in your gelatin mold, the longer it needs to set.

To store dried fruit, stir in enough flour to put in a covered container and place in the refrigerator.

Try sifting flour directly into the measuring cup and then level with the edge of a spatula.

When making pudding, it is the milk protein whey that burns at the bottom of the pan, and the skin that forms is casein, another protein. Place a piece of wax paper on top so water doesn't evaporate on top, forming a skin.

Fertile eggs result from the mating of a chicken and a rooster. Cooking the eggs shortly after they are laid prevents the natural hatching progression.

Test cakes by inserting a toothpick in the center. If it comes out dry, the cake is done.

Always preheat your oven before baking desserts -- or anything that requires accurate baking time.

It is advisable to keep cakes refrigerated that have cheese in the icing.

To sour milk add 1 Tablespoon lemon juice or vinegar to enough milk to make 1 cup.

The most difficult part of cooking is deciding what to cook!

Old Fashioned Apple Dumplings

2 cups flour
2 tsp. baking powder
1 tsp. salt
1/2 cup vegetable oil
2/3 cup low fat milk

Mix together to form a dough.
Roll out half of the dough.
Cut into 4 pieces - 2 times.

8 small apples, peeled and sliced
1/2 cup brown sugar
1/4 tsp. cinnamon
Dash nutmeg

Mix together for the filling.
Put a large spoonful with a dab of
margarine on each piece of dough.
Bring edges over the filling and seal.
Place in a loaf pan sprayed with non-
stick cooking spray.

1/2 cup butter or margarine
1-1/2 cups brown sugar
1-1/4 cups hot water
Dash nutmeg
Dash cinnamon

Mix together and bring to a boil to make
a sauce.

Pour sauce over dumplings.
Bake at 450°F for 10 minutes, then
reduce heat to 400°F for an additional
20 minutes.

Apple Crisp

8 large apples
2 cups raw oats
3/4 cup whole wheat pastry flour

Mix together.

1/2 cup margarine
1/3 cup honey

Melt and mix.
Add to the above mixture.

1 tsp. cinnamon
1/2 tsp. allspice
1/2 tsp. salt
1/4 cup pecans

Mix and add to the above ingredients.
Save a few sprinkles for topping.

Layer apples and filling in baking pan.
Bake at 375°F for 45 minutes.

Pumpkin Pie

3 cups pumpkin purée
3/4 cup honey
2 Tbsp. molasses
1/4 tsp. cloves
3 tsp. cinnamon
1-1/2 tsp. ginger
1/2 tsp. salt
4 eggs or egg substitute
1 can evaporated milk

Mix together and pour in pie crust or in buttered baking dish (with no pie crust).

Bake at 375°F for 30-40 minutes.

See pie crust recipes on pages 171-173.

Fresh Strawberry Pie

1-1/2 cups water
3/4 cup sugar
1/4 cup cornstarch
Pinch salt (optional)

Cook until thick and clear.
(Can cook in microwave, stirring every 60 seconds.)

1 pkg. strawberry gelatin

Add to the sauce and stir until dissolved. Cool.

1-1/4 quarts strawberries, sliced

Place in 2 cooked and cooled pie shells.
Pour cooled sauce over berries.
Chill in refrigerator until well set.

This same recipe can be used for other fresh fruit pies:

Peaches (sliced): use with peach or orange gelatin
Red Raspberries: use with red raspberry gelatin
Blueberries: use with black raspberry gelatin.

Lemon Pie

2 cups water
1 cup sugar
2 heaping Tbsp. cornstarch

Mix and cook until thick and clear.

1 lemon (juice and grated rind)
2 eggs or egg substitute

Add to the above sauce and cook one
more minute.
Cool and pour into baked pie shell.
Chill.

See our pie crust recipes on pages 171-173.

Meringue

2 egg whites
1/4 tsp. cream of tartar

In a small bowl, beat until frothy.

2 Tbsp. sugar

Beat sugar gradually into eggs.
Beat until stiff.

Swirl meringue on pie.
Bake at 375°F for 8-10 minutes.

Chocolate Strawberry Torte

22 oz. pkg. brownie mix, or make this quick one bowl chocolate cake

Line two 8 inch pans with wax paper or spray with non-stick cooking spray. Prepare mix as directed on package.

6 Tbsp. cocoa or carob
2 cups flour
1-1/2 cups sugar
1 tsp. baking soda
1 tsp. baking powder
1/8 tsp. salt

Sift together in large mixing bowl.

2 eggs or egg substitute
1/2 cup vegetable oil
1 cup cold water

Mix well.
Add at once to the above mixture.
Pour into pans that have been sprayed with non-stick cooking spray and lightly floured.
Bake at 350°F for 30-40 minutes.

Low fat filling

4 oz. light vanilla yogurt
4 oz. pkg. instant vanilla pudding
1/2 cup low fat milk

Whip in small bowl.
Chill for several minutes.

12 oz. low fat cottage cheese
2 Tbsp. sugar
1 tsp. vanilla

Place in blender.
Blend until very creamy.
Stir into the above ingredients.

1 quart fresh strawberries, hulled and sliced

When cool, place one cake layer on a serving plate.
Top with half of the pudding mixture and half of the berries.
Repeat another layer.
Refrigerate until ready to serve.

Regular filling

14 oz. sweetened condensed milk
1/2 cup cold water

Mix in large bowl.

4 oz. pkg. instant vanilla pudding

Beat into milk and water mixture. Chill 5 minutes.

14 oz. non-dairy whipped topping

Fold into pudding mixture.
Spread onto layers as directed.

Chocolate Cherry Torte

1 pkg. Swiss chocolate cake mix or
make this one bowl chocolate cake

Prepare as package directs.

6 Tbsp. cocoa or carob
2 cups flour
1-1/2 cups sugar
1 tsp. baking soda
1 tsp. baking powder
1/8 tsp. salt

Sift together in a large bowl.

2 eggs or egg substitute
1/2 cup vegetable oil
1 cup cold water

Add at once to the above.
Beat well.

Pour into two 8 inch cake pans sprayed
with non-stick cooking spray and floured.
Bake at 350°F for 30-40 minutes.

2 tsp. lemon juice
4 oz. light cream cheese
1 can light creamy vanilla frosting

Beat together.

21 oz. can cherry pie filling

When cake is cool, split layers by
pulling a white thread through them.

On each layer, spread some frosting mix
and pie filling.
Continue until each layer is stacked.
Finish with frosting and cherries on top.

Chill until ready to serve.

Strawberry Shortcut Cake

1 cup miniature marshmallows	Place in bottom of 9 x 13 inch pan that has been sprayed with non-stick cooking spray.
2 - 10 oz. pkgs. frozen strawberries (2 cups), thawed 3 oz. pkg. strawberry gelatin	Mix together. Set aside.
2-1/4 cups flour 1-1/2 cups sugar 1/2 cup vegetable oil 3 tsp. baking powder 1/2 tsp. salt 1 cup low fat milk 1 tsp. vanilla 3 eggs or egg substitute	Mix together in large bowl. Beat at medium speed for 3 minutes. Pour over marshmallows. Spoon strawberry mixture over batter. Bake at 350°F for 45-50 minutes. No icing required.

Old Fashioned Sugar Cookies

2 cups sugar 3/4 cup vegetable oil	Cream together.
2 eggs or egg substitute	Stir in the above mixture.
1 cup sour low fat milk 2 tsp. baking powder 1 tsp. baking soda Pinch salt 1 tsp. vanilla Dash nutmeg Dash cinnamon Flour to thicken	Add to the above ingredients. Mix well. May be dropped on a cookie sheet sprayed with non-stick cooking spray, or chill dough, roll out and cut in desired shapes. Bake at 375°F for 10-12 minutes.

Variations

1/2 cup drained crushed pineapple may be added to the above dough for a different flavor or some chopped nuts may be added.

Roll out 3-4 inch circles. On 1/2 put 1 teaspoon of your favorite jam. Fold over for a 1/2 circle, seal edges and bake.

Turtle Cake

1 pkg. chocolate cake mix 1/2 cup vegetable oil 1 cup light evaporated milk (from a 13 oz. can)	Blend together. Spread 1/2 of batter in 9 x 13 inch pan that has been sprayed with non-stick cooking spray and dusted with flour. Bake at 350°F for 15 minutes.
1 pkg. caramels	Melt caramels in remaining milk. Spread over warm cake.
1 cup semisweet chocolate chips 1 cup pecans, chopped	Sprinkle over cake. Pour on remaining batter. Bake another 15 minutes.

Raisin Apple Cake

3 cups unsifted flour 2 cups sugar 1 cup low fat mayonnaise 1/3 cup low fat milk 2 eggs or egg substitute 2 tsp. baking soda 1-1/2 tsp. cinnamon 1/2 tsp. nutmeg 1/2 tsp. salt 1/4 tsp. cloves	Mix all ingredients in a large mixing bowl. Beat at low speed 2 minutes.
3 cups apples, peeled and chopped 1 cup seedless raisins 1/2 cup walnuts, coarsely chopped (optional)	Stir into the above batter. Pour into a tube pan or two 8 inch layer pans that have been sprayed with non-stick cooking spray and dusted with flour. Bake at 350°F for 45 minutes.

If this cake is baked in a tube pan, dusting with powdered sugar is adequate for the topping.

Carob Torte

6 Tbsp. carob powder
2 cups flour
1-1/2 cups sugar
1 tsp. soda
1 tsp. baking powder
1/8 tsp. salt

Sift into large mixing bowl.

2 eggs or egg substitute
3/4 cup vegetable oil
1 cup cold water

Add all at once to the above ingredients.
Beat well.

Pour batter into two 8 inch layer pans
that have been sprayed with non-stick
cooking spray and sprinkled with flour.

Bake at 350°F for 35-40 minutes.

When cake is cool, split layers in half by
pulling a white thread through them,
making 4 layers.

Filling

8 oz. pkg. light cream cheese
12 oz. carton low fat cottage cheese,
  drained

Place in blender and blend very well.

2 tsp. vanilla
2/3 cup granulated sugar
1/3 cup carob powder

Add to the cheese mixture.
Blend very well.

Spread on each cake layer and stack.
Spread filling on sides of the tort.

The density of this cake makes it possible to slice very thin for each serving.

Carrot Cake

2 cups sugar	Blend together in a large mixing bowl.
4 eggs or egg substitute	
1-1/2 cups vegetable oil	
2 cups flour	Sift into the above mixture.
3 tsp. cinnamon	Beat well, about 2 minutes.
2 tsp. baking soda	
1 tsp. salt	
2 tsp. vanilla	
2 cups carrots, grated	Stir into the above ingredients.
1 cup pineapple, crushed	Pour into a 9 x 13 inch pan or two 8 inch layer pans that have been sprayed with non-stick cooking spray and dusted with flour.
	Bake in preheated 350°F oven for 45-60 minutes.

Icing

6 oz. light cream cheese	Place in a small mixing bowl.
1 cup powdered sugar	Mix until smooth and creamy.
1/2 cup flour	Add more sugar and flour if needed to get the consistency desired.
1 tsp. vanilla or 1 tsp. lemon juice	

Galliano Cake

2 cups flour
1 Tbsp. baking powder
1/2 cup vegetable oil
1 cup sugar
1/4 tsp. salt
4 oz. pkg. instant vanilla pudding
4 eggs or egg substitute
1/2 cup orange juice
1/2 cup galliano
1/2 cup low fat milk

Place all ingredients in a large mixing bowl.
Beat very well, about 2 minutes.

Pour batter into a bundt or tube pan that has been sprayed with non-stick cooking spray and sprinkled with flour.

Bake at 350°F for 50-60 minutes.
Cool 15 minutes, then turn upside down on serving plate to finish cooling. The cake should drop onto the plate as it cools.

When completely cool, dust with powdered sugar.

This cake is very dense and can be sliced very thin. It actually tastes better in thin slices. This is a very nice cake for the holidays, with red and green cherries used as decorations.

Rhubarb Crunch

1 cup flour
3/4 cup oatmeal
1/2 cup brown sugar, firmly packed
1/2 cup liquid margarine
1 tsp. cinnamon

Combine.
Press 1/2 mixture into a 9 x 13 inch pan sprayed with non-stick cooking spray.

4 cups rhubarb, diced

Place over crumbs.

3/4 cup sugar
2 Tbsp. cornstarch
1 cup water
1 tsp. vanilla

Combine and cook until thick.
Pour over rhubarb.
Top with remaining crumbs.

Bake at 300°F for 1 hour.

Spicy Banana Cupcakes

1 cup unbleached white flour 1 tsp. baking powder 1/2 tsp. salt	Mix together.
1/2 cup honey 1 Tbsp. margarine or vegetable oil 1 large banana, mashed 2 Tbsp. low fat milk 1 egg or egg substitute	Mix together and add to the dry ingredients. Bake in muffin cups at 350°F for 15 minutes; until golden brown.

Creamy Banana Frosting

1/2 cup powdered sugar 1 tsp. lemon juice 4 Tbsp. banana, mashed 3 Tbsp. margarine	Blend and spread on cooled cupcakes.

Fresh Peach Cobbler

1/2 cup water 1-1/2 Tbsp. cornstarch 1/3 cup brown sugar	Mix together. Cook until thick.
4 cups fresh peaches, sliced and sweetened 1 Tbsp. liquid margarine 1 Tbsp. lemon juice	Mix together and add to the above sauce. Pour into 8 inch round baking dish that has been sprayed with non-stick cooking spray.
1/2 cup flour 1/2 cup sugar 1/4 tsp. salt (optional) 1/2 tsp. baking powder 2 Tbsp. liquid margarine 1 egg or egg substitute, slightly beaten	Combine, beat and pour over the peach mixture. Bake at 400°F for 40-50 minutes.

Date Pudding

1 cup flour 1/3 cup sugar 2 tsp. baking powder 1 tsp. salt (optional)	Mix together.
1/2 cup milk 1/2 cup nuts, chopped 1 cup dates, cut up	Stir into the dry mixture. Spread into baking pan or dish.
3/4 cup water 3/4 cup orange juice 2/3 cup brown sugar, packed 3 Tbsp. liquid margarine	Bring to boil and pour over above mixture. Bake at 350°F for 50-55 minutes.

Bread Pudding

4 cups dry bread crumbs	Place in a baking dish that has been sprayed with non-stick cooking spray.
2 eggs or egg substitute, beaten 2 cups low fat milk 1/2 cup brown sugar Dash nutmeg Dash cinnamon	Mix ingredients. Pour over the bread. Let soak.
1/4 cup raisins or 1/4 cup dates, chopped (or use both)	Stir into the above mixture. Bake at 350°F for 30 minutes or until firm in the center.

Chocolate Nut Balls

1 cup vanilla wafers, crushed 1/3 cup pineapple juice	Mix together.
1 cup chocolate chips 2 Tbsp. margarine	Melt and stir until smooth. Pour into crumb mixture.
1/3 cup walnuts, chopped 1-1/2 cups powdered sugar	Add to the above mixture. Roll into balls.
Coconut	Sprinkle over balls. Cool slightly.

Molasses Drop Cookies

3/4 cup vegetable oil 1 cup sugar 1 cup molasses	Cream together.
2 eggs or egg substitute	Stir into the above mixture.
1 cup boiling water 1 Tbsp. baking soda 1/2 tsp. salt 2 tsp. ginger 2 tsp. cinnamon	Mix together. Add to the above ingredients. Mix well.
5 scant cups flour	Add slowly to dough. Mix well.
	Drop by spoonfuls onto a cookie sheet that has been sprayed with non-stick cooking spray.
	Bake at 400°F for 8-10 minutes.

Grandma's Ginger Snaps

1 cup sugar
1/2 cup vegetable oil

Cream together.

1 egg or egg substitute
1/4 cup molasses

Stir into the above mixture.

2 cups flour
2 level tsp. baking soda
1/2 tsp. salt
1 tsp. cinnamon
1/2 tsp. ginger
1/2 tsp. cloves

Sift together.
Add to the above ingredients.
Mix well.

Refrigerate dough 2 hours or longer.

Form dough into balls (about size of quarters).
Roll in sugar.
Place on cookie sheets sprayed with non-stick cooking spray.

DO NOT flatten.

Bake at 375°F for 8-10 minutes.

Light Fruit Whip

3/4 cup cold water
1/4 cup powdered milk

Place in a medium size mixing bowl.
Beat until fluffy.

Gelatin - any flavor desired

Prepare as directed on the package.
Refrigerate until it begins to set.
Beat with electric mixer until fluffy.

Fold into milk mixture.
Put in serving dishes.
Chill until ready to serve.

This is a very light tasty dessert.

Lemon Bisque

1 pkg. lemon gelatin 1-1/4 cups boiling water Juice and rind of 1 lemon 1/2 cup sugar	Mix and chill until syrupy. Beat with electric mixer until fluffy.
1 large can low fat evaporated milk, chilled 1 tsp. vanilla Dash salt (optional) 3 Tbsp. sugar	Beat until fluffy. Fold into the above mixture.
1 cup graham cracker crumbs	Place crumbs in the bottom of a deep pie plate or square dish and pour in lemon mixture. Chill until well set. Cut into squares and serve.

Orange Soufflé

2 Tbsp. cornstarch 2 Tbsp. sugar	Combine in aluminum saucepan.
3/4 cup low fat evaporated milk 3 Tbsp. undiluted orange juice concentrate, thawed 2 Tbsp. low sugar orange marmalade 1 tsp. vanilla extract	Add to above. Cook, stirring constantly with whisk, until thick. Place in large bowl. Set aside to cool.
6 egg whites 1/2 tsp. cream of tartar	Beat until stiff, but not dry. Stir 1/4 meringue into milk mixture. Fold in remaining meringue. Spoon mixture into 2 quart soufflé dish that has been sprayed with non-stick cooking spray. Bake at 425°F for 1 minute, then at 375°F for 25 minutes. Serve immediately.

Cinnamon Sticks

1 dozen

2 large egg whites	Beat until peaks form.
1/2 cup sugar	Slowly add to eggs.
1 cup unbleached white flour 1 tsp. cinnamon	Stir into egg mixture.
1/3 cup margarine or vegetable oil	Add to above ingredients.
	Spray cookie sheet with non-stick cooking spray. Spoon 2 measuring teaspoonfuls batter onto cookie sheet. Press with back of spoon and make a 3 inch flat circle. Bake at 350°F for 6 minutes. While still warm, use a wooden spoon and roll up cookies around spoon. Slide cookie off spoon. Let cool.

Rum Balls

1 cup semisweet chocolate pieces	Melt and remove from heat.
1/4 cup sugar 3 Tbsp. honey 1/3 cup rum	Stir into melted chocolate.
2-1/2 cups vanilla wafers, finely chopped 1/3 cup walnuts, chopped	Add to above mixture. Shape into 1 inch balls. Roll in powdered sugar if desired. Refrigerate.

Fudge Cookies

1 dozen

6 oz. unsweetened chocolate or powdered carob 1 Tbsp. vegetable oil	Melt chocolate. Remove from heat.
2 cups unbleached white flour 2 tsp. baking powder	Mix together.
1 cup sugar 1/2 cup vegetable oil 2 Tbsp. low fat milk 2 tsp. vanilla 3 medium eggs or egg substitute	Mix together and add to melted chocolate. Add dry ingredients. Refrigerate 1 hour. Place on oiled cookie sheet in 1-inch balls and flatten. Bake at 375°F for 10 minutes. Let cool.

Apricot Twisties

1 dozen

1/3 cup apricot preserves 1/3 cup honey 1/4 cup water 1/4 tsp. vanilla	Mix together.
2 cups unbleached white flour 1/4 tsp. baking powder 1/2 tsp. vanilla 1/2 tsp. salt	Mix together.
1/2 cup margarine	Cut into dry ingredients. Stir into apricot mixture. Roll out dough 1/4 inch thick and 1 inch wide. Twist each strip and place on cookie sheet. Bake at 375°F for 10 minutes. Sprinkle with powdered sugar.

Cappuccino Cookies

1-1/2 dozen

1/2 cup margarine	Beat until soft.
1/2 cup sugar 1/3 cup brown sugar	Add to softened margarine. Beat until fluffy.
2 oz. unsweetened chocolate, melted 1 Tbsp. instant coffee, dissolved in 1 Tbsp. water 2 eggs or egg substitute	Add to above mixture. Mix well.
2 cups unbleached white flour 1 tsp. cinnamon 1/4 tsp. salt	Add to above ingredients. Place by spoonfuls on baking sheet. Flatten slightly. Can sprinkle with crushed almonds. Bake at 350°F for 12 minutes.

Marzipan Squares

12 squares

8 oz. almond paste 1/2 cup margarine	Cream together in blender.
3 eggs or egg substitute 1 cup sugar	Add slowly to blender.
2 cups unbleached white flour 1 tsp. baking powder	Mix together.
1 cup low fat milk	Add slowly to blender with flour mixture. Spray baking pans with non-stick cooking spray. Spread batter into pan. Bake at 350°F for 45 minutes. Let cool, then cut into small squares.

Cherry Cookies

3 dozen

1/2 cup margarine 1/2 cup sugar 1/4 cup honey 1 egg or egg substitute 1-1/2 tsp. vanilla	Beat together until fluffy.
1-1/4 cups unbleached white flour 1/4 cup cocoa or carob powder 1/4 tsp. baking powder 1/4 tsp. baking soda 1/4 tsp. salt	Mix together. Slowly add to above ingredients.
10 oz. jar maraschino cherries, finely chopped	Add to dough. Shape dough into 1 inch balls and lightly press to shape. Bake at 350°F for 10 minutes.

Almond Custard

Serves 4

1 envelope unflavored gelatin 5 Tbsp. water	Mix together in saucepan. Cook over low heat until gelatin is dissolved.
1-1/4 cups vanilla low fat yogurt 1/3 cup honey 1 egg or egg substitute 1/2 tsp. almond extract	Mix together in blender until smooth. Add heated gelatin and blend. Place in custard cups. Chill until set. Sprinkle with cinnamon and almond slices.

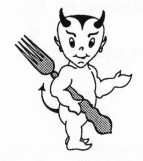

16. Making a Good Cup of Coffee

Do you stagger out of bed and straight to the coffee maker each morning? Does the thought of drinking a cup of coffee made at your office make you cringe? Have faith -- anyone can make a great cup of coffee.

Coffee is like a fine wine, and there are many species of coffee plants. The best quality Arabica beans come from Columbia where the soil, weather and high elevation create ideal conditions. Columbian is a full-bodied coffee. Another commonly used bean is Robusta, which is grown primarily in Africa at low altitudes, and is less expensive than Columbian -- but lacks the flavor and richness. Robusta beans also contains twice as much caffeine as Arabica and are used in most instant coffees.

Be creative and make your own blend by combining several different coffees.

Selecting a Bean

We want you to enjoy your cup of coffee -- while drinking it in MODERATION. So why not drink one cup of coffee with a rich and superb flavor -- instead of drinking 5 cups of old stale bitter coffee?

Sumatra is grown primarily in southeast Asia and has a wine-like taste. It is a high quality coffee with a superb flavor.

Kona is grown in Hawaii and has a full-bodied and sweet flavor.

Colombian has a full-bodied flavor with a slightly smoky flavor and is similar to Guatemalan coffee.

Jamaican has a delicious delicate flavor like mountain coffee.

Indonesian has a superb spicy taste and is high quality coffee.

Mexican has an excellent high quality coffee "Altura," which has a spicy full-bodied flavor.

French or Continental roast - It is the roasting that brings out the aroma and flavor of the bean. This roasting method is a dark brown roast that produces a tangy flavor with an oily surface.

Regular roast is a medium brown roast and has a sweet and rich flavor. It is the basic roast used in most coffee.

Grinding and Storage

Coffee beans, if not stored properly in an airtight container in the freezer, can become stale fast. Keep your beans about 6 weeks, and buy small amounts at a time. It's best to grind beans just before brewing. If your coffee tastes bitter or too strong, your grind may be too fine or you used too much coffee. If it lacks flavor, your grind may be too coarse or you need more coffee.

Measuring and Brewing Coffee

Try using two level tablespoons of coffee for each 6 oz. cup. When brewing, some people use tap water or spring water to give coffee its fullest flavor. Softener water can add a salty taste to coffee and distilled water leaves a flat taste because minerals have been removed.

Try not to overbrew and serve as soon as it is ready. Reheating coffee gives it a great flavor. Percolators should be avoided -- they will repeatedly boil and cook the coffee making it bitter by bringing out the tannic acid in the bean. Take your leftover coffee and pour it into a THERMOS; this will keep it from getting bitter.

Caffeine and Decaffeination

Moderation is the key. Caffeine isn't bad, but when you continue to nervously pour down cup-after-cup and your heart is racing -- it is now an unhealthful beverage. Just like drinking too much soda or tea, etc...

Decaffeinated coffee still contains small amounts of caffeine -- about 4 milligrams in a 5 ounce cup. Regular brewed coffee has approximately 65-120 milligrams in a 5 ounce cup. Most coffees are decaffeinated by using the solvent, "ethyl acetate" or another method, "Swiss Water Process." Both are FDA approved. Read your labels and make sure the company that makes your decaffeinated coffee is not using "methylene chloride," which could be a health hazard.

Coffee Substitutes

Chicory is the most commonly used substitute for coffee. It is a plant that has a root -- with a coffee like flavor when ground. Another substitute is roasted barley, which has a unique and good tasting coffee flavor.

Index

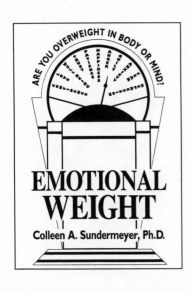

A Great Gift!

Eat No Evil Apron

"There are no bad, evil or forbidden foods"

Bon Appetit!

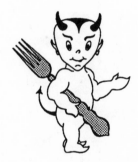 We want you to have fun in the kitchen. Therefore, we have designed an apron for you.

The apron is made with white twill fabric and red contrasting binding trim with a center-stitched bottom pouch. The fabric is 50% polyester/50% cotton; 17 x 21 inches. Our little devil is the two color printed silk screen design on the front center.

Style #2035 Custom Manufacturer
Manufacturer's Suggested Retail Price

$16.95 plus $2.25 shipping and handling.

Send check or money order to:

New Outlook
6373 Riverside Boulevard
Box 114
Sacramento, CA 95831
(916)395-8010

Allow 2-4 weeks for delivery.